THE CTSA PROGRAM AT NIH

Opportunities for Advancing Clinical
and Translational Research

Committee to Review the Clinical and Translational Science
Awards Program at the National Center for Advancing
Translational Sciences

Board on Health Sciences Policy

Alan I. Leshner, Sharon F. Terry, Andrea M. Schultz
and Catharyn T. Liverman, *Editors*

INSTITUTE OF MEDICINE
OF THE NATIONAL ACADEMIES

THE NATIONAL ACADEMIES PRESS
Washington, D.C.
www.nap.edu

THE NATIONAL ACADEMIES PRESS • 500 Fifth Street, NW • Washington, DC 20001

NOTICE: The project that is the subject of this report was approved by the Governing Board of the National Research Council, whose members are drawn from the councils of the National Academy of Sciences, the National Academy of Engineering, and the Institute of Medicine.

This project was supported by a contract between the National Academy of Sciences and the National Institutes of Health (Award No. HHSN26300001). The views presented in this publication are those of the editors and attributing authors and do not necessarily reflect the view of the organizations or agencies that provided support for this project.

International Standard Book Number-13: 978-0-309-28474-5
International Standard Book Number-10: 0-309-28474-0

Additional copies of this report available for sale from the National Academies Press, 500 Fifth Street, NW, Keck 360, Washington, DC 20001; (800) 624-6242 or (202) 334-3313; http://www.nap.edu.

For more information about the Institute of Medicine, visit the IOM home page at: **www.iom.edu.**

Suggested citation: IOM (Institute of Medicine). 2013. *The CTSA Program at NIH: Opportunities for advancing clinical and translational research.* Washington, DC: The National Academies Press.

"Knowing is not enough; we must apply.
Willing is not enough; we must do."
—Goethe

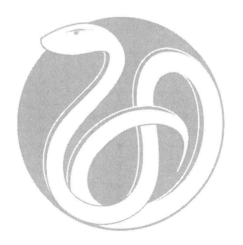

INSTITUTE OF MEDICINE
OF THE NATIONAL ACADEMIES

Advising the Nation. Improving Health.

THE NATIONAL ACADEMIES
Advisers to the Nation on Science, Engineering, and Medicine

The **National Academy of Sciences** is a private, nonprofit, self-perpetuating society of distinguished scholars engaged in scientific and engineering research, dedicated to the furtherance of science and technology and to their use for the general welfare. Upon the authority of the charter granted to it by the Congress in 1863, the Academy has a mandate that requires it to advise the federal government on scientific and technical matters. Dr. Ralph J. Cicerone is president of the National Academy of Sciences.

The **National Academy of Engineering** was established in 1964, under the charter of the National Academy of Sciences, as a parallel organization of outstanding engineers. It is autonomous in its administration and in the selection of its members, sharing with the National Academy of Sciences the responsibility for advising the federal government. The National Academy of Engineering also sponsors engineering programs aimed at meeting national needs, encourages education and research, and recognizes the superior achievements of engineers. Dr. C. D. Mote, Jr., is president of the National Academy of Engineering.

The **Institute of Medicine** was established in 1970 by the National Academy of Sciences to secure the services of eminent members of appropriate professions in the examination of policy matters pertaining to the health of the public. The Institute acts under the responsibility given to the National Academy of Sciences by its congressional charter to be an adviser to the federal government and, upon its own initiative, to identify issues of medical care, research, and education. Dr. Harvey V. Fineberg is president of the Institute of Medicine.

The **National Research Council** was organized by the National Academy of Sciences in 1916 to associate the broad community of science and technology with the Academy's purposes of furthering knowledge and advising the federal government. Functioning in accordance with general policies determined by the Academy, the Council has become the principal operating agency of both the National Academy of Sciences and the National Academy of Engineering in providing services to the government, the public, and the scientific and engineering communities. The Council is administered jointly by both Academies and the Institute of Medicine. Dr. Ralph J. Cicerone and Dr. C. D. Mote, Jr., are chair and vice chair, respectively, of the National Research Council.

www.national-academies.org

COMMITTEE TO REVIEW THE CLINICAL AND TRANSLATIONAL SCIENCE AWARDS PROGRAM AT THE NATIONAL CENTER FOR ADVANCING TRANSLATIONAL SCIENCES

ALAN I. LESHNER (*Chair*), American Association for the Advancement of Science, Washington, DC
SHARON F. TERRY (*Vice-Chair*), Genetic Alliance, Washington, DC
SUSAN AXELROD, Citizens United for Research in Epilepsy, Chicago, IL
ENRIQUETA C. BOND, Burroughs Wellcome Fund (*Emeritus*), Marshall, VA
ANN C. BONHAM, Association of American Medical Colleges, Washington, DC
SUSAN J. CURRY, University of Iowa, Iowa City
PHYLLIS A. DENNERY, University of Pennsylvania, Philadelphia
RALPH I. HORWITZ, GlaxoSmithKline, King of Prussia, PA
JEFFREY P. KAHN, Johns Hopkins University, Baltimore, MD
ROBIN T. KELLEY, National Minority AIDS Council, Washington, DC
MARGARET McCABE, Boston Children's Hospital, MA
EDITH A. PEREZ, Mayo Clinic, Jacksonville, FL
CLIFFORD J. ROSEN, Maine Medical Center Research Institute, Scarborough

IOM Staff

CATHARYN T. LIVERMAN, Study Director
ANDREA M. SCHULTZ, Study Director
MARGARET A. McCOY, Program Officer (*beginning March 2013*)
CLAIRE F. GIAMMARIA, Research Associate
JUDITH L. ESTEP, Program Associate
ANDREW M. POPE, Director, Board on Health Sciences Policy

Consultant

VICTORIA WEISFELD, Technical Writer

Reviewers

This report has been reviewed in draft form by individuals chosen for their diverse perspectives and technical expertise, in accordance with procedures approved by the National Research Council's Report Review Committee. The purpose of this independent review is to provide candid and critical comments that will assist the institution in making its published report as sound as possible and to ensure that the report meets institutional standards for objectivity, evidence, and responsiveness to the study charge. The review comments and draft manuscript remain confidential to protect the integrity of the deliberative process. We wish to thank the following individuals for their review of this report:

Gordon R. Bernard, Vanderbilt University
Wylie Burke, University of Washington
Jonathan Davis, Tufts University School of Medicine
Jaqueline B. Fine, Merck Research Laboratories
Garret A. FitzGerald, University of Pennsylvania School of Medicine
Robert C. Gallo, University of Maryland School of Medicine
Margaret Grey, Yale University School of Nursing
Kevin Grumbach, University of California, San Francisco
William N. Kelley, University of Pennsylvania School of Medicine
Michael D. Lairmore, University of California, Davis
Elizabeth O. Ofili, Morehouse School of Medicine
Bray Patrick-Lake, Clinical Trials Transformation Initiative
Doris Rubio, University of Pittsburgh

Although the reviewers listed above have provided many constructive comments and suggestions, they did not see the final draft of the report before its release. The review of this report was overseen by **Floyd E. Bloom,** The Scripps Research Institute. Appointed by the Institute of Medicine, he was responsible for making certain that an independent examination of this report was carried out in accordance with institutional procedures and that all review comments were carefully considered. Responsibility for the final content of this report rests entirely with the authoring committee and the institution.

Preface

Private- and public-sector investment in health care is immense, and wide agreement exists in both sectors that the U.S. health care system needs to be improved in many ways in order to reduce costs and provide equitable access to high-quality care. The availability of cutting-edge technologies and new preventive and therapeutic interventions is a result of the United States' historic investment in biomedical and health research. New efforts in clinical and translational research hold great promise for even more effective and efficient ways to improve the health of our population. Investments in research support tools, informatics, infrastructure, and training and education are essential to facilitate new discoveries and to move promising discoveries in basic science and clinical research into use in clinics, hospitals, and homes.

In 2006, the National Institutes of Health (NIH) began an investment in the Clinical and Translational Science Awards (CTSA) Program, a bold initiative aimed at facilitating and accelerating clinical and translational research—lofty and challenging goals. Simultaneously building on a legacy program (NIH's General Clinical Research Center Program) and pioneering a new initiative is never easy.

Our Institute of Medicine (IOM) committee was given the task of assessing progress and recommending a path forward to help improve the efficiency and effectiveness of one of the nation's most important resources for clinical and translational science. As we assessed the CTSA Program, we were fully cognizant of both the importance of our task and the opportunity it presented. Among our conclusions was that the CTSA Program has had many initial successes in creating academic homes for clinical and translational research, providing education and training, and beginning to build the tools and partnerships needed to advance clinical and translational science. As requested by the sponsor, we identified ways the program can be strengthened.

The future of the CTSA Program is exciting, as well as daunting. Although there is great potential for the creation of new preventive and treatment approaches, there remain numerous institutional, logistical, and methodological barriers to doing so. Moving clinical and translational research forward will greatly benefit from the strong leadership, creative partnerships, and institutional commitments that the CTSA Program can bring to this effort.

It was our pleasure and privilege to lead the efforts of this IOM committee—superb committee members and outstanding staff who have worked diligently to learn about this complex program and contemplate the potential for its future. The expertise and grace of these generous individuals combined to create deep discourse and solid consensus.

We thank everyone who provided testimony, gave presentations, and participated in discussions with the committee. We are grateful to the staff of the National Center for Advancing Translational Sciences (NCATS) who responded thoroughly to our numerous inquiries. The committee is truly appreciative of the many individuals who provided the diversity and breadth of knowledge and opinion needed to complete this study.

The CTSA Program has made some remarkable progress to date and has great potential to further advance clinical and translational science and improve human health. We look forward to seeing this potential fully realized in the coming years.

Alan I. Leshner, *Chair*
Sharon F. Terry, *Vice-Chair*
Committee to Review the Clinical and
Translational Science Awards Program at the
National Center for Advancing Translational Sciences

Contents

Summary

During the past half-century, biomedical research has expanded exponentially, yielding many discoveries that offer the promise of improved human health. Translating basic and clinical research findings into clinical and community practice has been slow and cumbersome, however, and many years may pass before the benefits of research reach individual patients and communities. Recognizing the need for a new impetus to spur clinical and translational research, the National Institutes of Health (NIH) established the Clinical and Translational Science Awards (CTSA) Program in 2006.

The CTSA Program was designed to "provide integrated intellectual and physical resources for the conduct of original clinical and translational science,"[1] and individual CTSA sites were intended to serve as "catalysts and test beds for policies and practices that can benefit clinical and translational research organizations throughout the country."[2] In its first 7 years, the CTSA Program grew from 12 initial sites to the current 61, which are housed at academic health centers and other institutions across the United States. During this time, the program has made notable strides in accomplishing its initial goal of reshaping clinical and translational research at these institutions and has begun to build a national network that has the potential to catalyze further progress.

In 2012 the NIH contracted with the Institute of Medicine (IOM) to conduct a consensus study to assess and provide recommendations on the

---

[1]Zerhouni, E. A. 2005. Translational and clinical science—time for a new vision. *New England Journal of Medicine* 353(15):1621–1623.

[2]Zerhouni, E. A. 2006. Clinical and Translational Science Awards: A framework for a national research agenda. *Translational Research* 148(1):4–5.

appropriateness of the CTSA Program's mission and strategic goals and whether changes were needed. The committee was also tasked with providing an independent appraisal of and advice on the implementation of the program by the National Center for Advancing Translational Sciences (NCATS), while exploring the contributions of CTSAs in accelerating the development of new therapeutics, facilitating disease-specific and child health research, and enhancing the integration of research funded by NIH institutes and centers. To conduct this study, the IOM convened a 13-member committee with expertise in community outreach and engagement, public health and health policy, bioethics, education and training, pharmaceutical research and development, program evaluation, clinical and biomedical research, and child health research, along the full continuum of clinical and translation research. The committee's overarching conclusion is that the CTSA Program is contributing significantly to the advancement of clinical and translational research and is therefore a worthwhile investment that would benefit from a variety of revisions to make it more efficient and effective.

THE CTSA PROGRAM

The CTSA Program is a direct outgrowth of the NIH's General Clinical Research Center Program, which for more than 40 years provided clinical research infrastructure funding. Development of the CTSA Program was an integral part of the implementation of the 2004 *NIH Roadmap for Medical Research*. From 2006 to 2011, the program was administered through the NIH's National Center for Research Resources. In fiscal year (FY) 2012, NIH established NCATS, and the CTSA Program became the largest component of that center.

Individual CTSAs are funded through 5-year cooperative agreements, and site budgets range from $4 million to $23 million annually, with a total CTSA Program budget of $461 million in FY2012. Building an active and productive CTSA at an institution often involves not only the funds from the CTSA cooperative agreement but also substantial financial and staff commitments from the institution; although institutional cost sharing is not required. The committee could not identify any data to quantify these institutional contributions but heard testimony from many individuals about the depth of efforts and the commitment to the CTSA Program from top leaders at health research institutions across the nation.

Currently the 61 CTSAs provide a wide array of training and research support to help researchers identify promising therapeutics and interventions and move them forward as rapidly as possible. Research support is provided in areas that include core facilities; biomedical informatics; pilot funding; regulatory knowledge and support; biostatistics, epidemiology, research design, and ethics; participant and clinical interaction resources; and community engagement efforts and resources.

From the outset of the program, the NIH charged the CTSAs with developing a national consortium to promote the identification and use of best research practices. This effort has developed into the primarily self-governing CTSA Consortium, which oversees numerous collaborative committees. The CTSA Consortium's efforts are guided by three leadership committees: an Executive Committee, a Steering Committee, and a Child Health Oversight Committee. In addition, CTSA principal investigators, researchers, and staff work on 5 strategic goal committees and 14 key function committees (plus a number of interest groups, task forces, and work groups) that were established over time to discuss crosscutting issues, promote collaboration, and identify and implement best practices.

In November 2011, the CTSA Consortium Coordinating Center was established at Vanderbilt University through a competitive application process. The coordinating center has taken many steps to standardize and coordinate consortium activities and is working to ensure the availability of best practices, facilitate the uptake of available tools and resources, and promote collaboration, in part through its website, CTSACentral.org.

CONTEXT AND VISION FOR THE CTSA PROGRAM

The CTSA Program does not exist in isolation; it is part of a larger clinical and translational research ecosystem that plays a vital role in an increasingly complex and dynamic U.S. health care system. Decades of innovation and technological advances have led to progress in biomedical sciences, medicine, and public health, contributing to increased life expectancy and improved individual and population health. At the same time, however, the accelerating pace of scientific discoveries has also been one cause of the increasing complexity of the U.S. health care system, contributing to inconsistent health care quality and escalating costs.

Across the United States, momentum is growing in support of a learning health care system in which researchers and health care providers design and implement care, evaluations, or research based on needs of specific communities and populations. The findings are disseminated to inform clinical practice and research models to improve health. A learning health care system is founded on the concept of continuous improvement and the imperative to translate "what we know" into "what we do." Such a system fuels greater value in health care by harnessing the promise of new technological capabilities, market opportunities, and policies. Thus, clinical and translational research is integral to a learning health care system.

The CTSA Program has been successful in establishing CTSAs as academic focal points for clinical and translational research. The challenge for the next phase of the program—which NCATS has described as CTSA 2.0—will be to set the goals and create incentives for its 61 sites to function as the core of a national network that initiates and sustains collaborations both inside and outside their home institutions; across NIH institutes and centers; and with community, industry, and research network partners. The IOM committee envisions a transformation of the CTSA Program from its current, loosely organized structure into a more tightly integrated network that works collectively to enhance the transit of therapeutics, diagnostics, and preventive interventions along the developmental pipeline; disseminate innovative translational research methods and best practices; and provide leadership in informatics standards and policy development to promote shared resources.

The committee identified four key opportunities for action:

- *Adopt and sustain active program leadership*—NCATS should increase its leadership presence in the overall program, consistent with the cooperative agreement model under which the CTSAs are funded. A centralized leadership model that includes participation by NCATS, leaders of individual CTSAs, community partners, and other stakeholders will increase overall program efficiency, enable mechanisms for maximizing accountability, and provide the direction needed to develop and nurture substantive partnerships.

- *Engage in substantive and productive collaborations*—The CTSA Program needs to capitalize on the collaborations developed within and among individual CTSAs and continue to initiate and forge true partnerships with other NIH institutes and centers and with entities external to the program, including patient groups, communities, health care providers, industry, and regulatory organizations.

- *Develop and widely disseminate innovative research resources*—Fully developing the role of the CTSA Program as a facilitator and accelerator of clinical and translational research will require enhanced efforts to engage and support researchers and other stakeholders as they develop, refine, widely disseminate, and implement novel research and health informatics tools, methodologies, policies, and other resources.

- *Build on initial successes in training and education, community engagement, and child health research*—The CTSA Program needs to continue its strong efforts in each of these areas. A robust and diverse workforce that is well trained in team science is critically important. Ensuring an emphasis on community involvement across the research spectrum will bring a range of much-needed perspectives and innovations along with increased public support for research. Program efforts can also help overcome the paucity of research specific to child health.

LEADERSHIP

Today's CTSA Program has a complex, multilevel structure of organization and oversight involving NCATS, individual CTSAs, the CTSA Consortium with multiple levels and type of committees and working groups, and the CTSA Coordinating Center. An initiative with the scope and structure of the CTSA Program inherently faces challenges in balancing grassroots and top-down leadership approaches. To date, the program has, for the most part, relied on the energy and efforts of individual CTSAs and their principal investigators. As the program moves forward, the IOM committee sees the need for a more centralized approach to leadership, one in which NCATS plays a much more active role.

The IOM committee envisions the primary governance of the program residing within a new NCATS-CTSA Steering Committee that would be responsible for program oversight and direction; trans-CTSA activities; collaborative efforts with external partners; promotion of collaborative opportunities within and outside of NIH; identification, dissemination, and implementation of best practices; and implementation of a proposed new innovations fund to promote collaboration with other NIH institutes and centers and external partners.

A strategic planning process is needed as NCATS leads the program into its next phase. The program's mission statement should be updated to clarify its overall purpose and to align it with the mission of NCATS. Identifying and disseminating a set of clearly defined, measurable strategic goals is the starting point for shaping the program's future. These measurable goals should serve as a foundation for developing high-level common metrics and measures that could be applied and publicly reported on consistently to demonstrate progress. At this point, NCATS's plans for evaluating individual CTSA sites and the CTSA Program as a whole are unclear. Progress is being made at the individual CTSA level in terms of self-evaluation, but the current lack of transparency in reporting and lack of high-level common metrics are barriers to overall program accountability.

Streamlining the current consortium structure is an urgent need. However, the structure and governance should evolve during the next year or two as a component of the recommended strategic planning process. Only those consortium committees that are most relevant to the program's revised goals and priorities should be retained.

Recommendation 1: *Strengthen NCATS Leadership of the CTSA Program*

NCATS should strengthen its leadership of the CTSA Program to advance innovative and transformative efforts in clinical and translational research. As it implements CTSA 2.0, NCATS should

- **increase active involvement in the CTSA cooperative agreements and the CTSA Consortium;**
- **conduct a strategic planning process to set measurable goals and objectives for the program that address the full spectrum of clinical and translational research;**
- **ensure that the CTSA Program as a whole actively supports the full spectrum of clinical and translational research while encouraging flexibility for each institution to build on its unique strengths;**
- **form strategic partnerships with NIH institutes and centers and with other research networks and industry;**
- **establish an innovations fund through a set-aside mechanism that would be used for collaborative pilot studies and other initiatives involving CTSA institutions, other NIH institutes, and/or other public and private entities (e.g., industry, other**

government agencies, private foundations, community advocates and organizations);

- evaluate the program as a whole to identify gaps, weaknesses, and opportunities and create mechanisms to address them; and
- distill and widely disseminate best practices and lessons learned by the CTSA Program and work to communicate its value and accomplishments and seek opportunities for further efforts and collaborations.

Recommendation 2: *Reconfigure and Streamline the CTSA Consortium*

NCATS should reconfigure and streamline the structure of the CTSA Program by establishing a new multistakeholder NCATS-CTSA Steering Committee that would

- be chaired by a member of NCATS leadership team and have a CTSA principal investigator as vice-chair, and
- provide direction to the CTSA Coordinating Center in developing and promoting the use of available shared resources.

Recommendation 3: *Build on the Strengths of Individual CTSAs Across the Spectrum of Clinical and Translational Research*

Individual CTSAs, with the leadership of NCATS, should emphasize their particular strengths in advancing the program's broad mission and goals. In doing so, CTSAs should

- drive innovation and collaboration in methodologies, processes, tools, and resources across the spectrum of clinical and translational research;
- emphasize interdisciplinary team-based approaches in training, education, and research;
- involve patients, family members, health care providers, and other community partners in all phases of the work of the CTSA;
- strengthen collaborations across the schools and disciplines in their home institutions;

- build partnerships with industry, other research networks, community groups, and other stakeholders; and
- communicate the resources available through the CTSA Program.

Recommendation 4: *Formalize and Standardize Evaluation Processes for Individual CTSAs and the CTSA Program*

NCATS should formalize and standardize its evaluation processes for individual CTSAs and the CTSA Program. The evaluations should use clear, consistent, and innovative metrics that align with the program's mission and goals and that go beyond standard academic benchmarks of publications and number of grant awards to assess the CTSA Program and the individual CTSAs.

CROSSCUTTING TOPICS

The CTSA Program has demonstrated progress in three crosscutting domains that the IOM committee believes are integral to advancing clinical and translational science effectively: training and education, community engagement, and child health research. These efforts, along with the program's contributions in building infrastructure and providing a range of research resources, make the CTSA Program a unique national resource within the clinical and translational research landscape. Each of these functions can be strengthened, as discussed below.

Training and Education

Sustaining a vibrant clinical and translational research enterprise in the future depends on building and retaining a diverse research workforce. Education and training in clinical and translational research are priorities for the CTSA Program. All CTSA institutions are expected to provide robust postgraduate training, and many have extensive training programs that include undergraduate and predoctoral student training as well as training for research staff and community collaborators. The KL2 and TL1 training awards[3] have been an integral part of CTSA training programs. In FY2011, 501 scholars participated in the KL2 program, and 469 trainees participated in the TL1 program through the CTSA Program. Moving forward, the committee urges increased flexibility in training and education programs with options available to personalize the training experience to meet the needs and goals of individual participants.

This flexibility will be valuable in attracting and retaining scholars and trainees and may be particularly pertinent to the clinician-scientists who are essential in clinical and translational research. NCATS and individual CTSAs have the opportunity to lead changes in the following: emphasizing the team-based skills that are required in clinical and translational research, developing metrics to assess clinical and translational training and education programs, and instituting incentives for recognition and promotion of those involved. New benchmarks that value team-based efforts and collaborative approaches are needed to complement the traditional benchmarks for academic success that focus on individual accomplishments and products (e.g., publications, new grants).

Recommendation 5: *Advance Innovation in Education and Training Programs*

The CTSA Program should provide training, mentoring, and education as essential core elements. To better prepare the next generation of a diverse clinical and translational science workforce, the CTSA Program should

- **emphasize innovative education and training models and methodologies, which include a focus on team science, leadership, community engagement, and entrepreneurship;**
- **disseminate high-quality online offerings for essential core courses for use in CTSA and other institutions;**

---

[3]The KL2 Mentored Clinical Research Scholar Program is a career development award that provides individuals who have a doctoral degree with formal research experience and funding support to help them become independent investigators in clinical and translational research. The TL1 Clinical Research Training Program provides an introduction to clinical and translational research to pre- and postdoctoral candidates or others who want to learn more about these types of research.

- champion the reshaping of career development pathways for researchers involved in the conduct of clinical and translational science; and
- ensure flexible and personalized training experiences that offer optional advanced degrees.

Community Engagement

The ultimate goal of translational research—to improve human health—requires meaningful community engagement across the entire spectrum of research from basic science to community and population health research. Communities can contribute to the full range of clinical and translational research in important ways that are not always recognized. For example, partnerships with community representatives can identify community health needs and priorities, provide critical input and data on clinically relevant questions, develop culturally appropriate clinical research protocols, promote successful enrollment and retention of research participants, and, ultimately, disseminate and implement research results more effectively.

The initial commitment to community engagement within the CTSA Program should be commended. However, NCATS's vision for how community engagement will be a part of the CTSA Program moving forward remains unclear. Although indications point to community engagement remaining an important feature of the program, there are serious concerns that if it is not an explicit requirement for all CTSAs, it may fade in importance. The IOM committee fully supports community engagement and involvement throughout the entire research process and believes that this program component is essential and needs to be preserved, nurtured, and expanded.

Because involving the community in the continuum of research is a new experience for many researchers, the CTSA Program and NCATS must provide clear guidance and leadership that effectively define and communicate goals and expectations.

Recommendation 6: *Ensure Community Engagement in All Phases of Research*

NCATS and the CTSA Program should ensure that patients, family members, health care providers, clinical researchers, and

other community stakeholders are involved across the continuum of clinical and translational research. NCATS and the CTSA Program should

- define community engagement broadly and use this definition consistently in requests for applications and communications about the CTSA Program;
- ensure active and substantive community stakeholder participation in priority setting and decision making across all phases of clinical and translational research and in the leadership and governance of the CTSA Program;
- define and clearly communicate goals and expectations for community engagement at the individual CTSA level and across the program and ensure the broad dissemination of best practices in community engagement; and
- explore opportunities and incentives to engage a more diverse community.

Child Health Research

For too long, research examining the safety and efficacy of medications and other health interventions has focused on adults, and little has been known about health- and development-related impacts of medications, devices, and preventive measures on children. Thus, clinical and translational research is urgently needed in the area of child health. The IOM committee believes that the CTSA Program has placed an appropriate emphasis on accelerating clinical and translational research to improve child health, and the CTSA Program, through the CTSA Consortium Child Health Oversight Committee (CC-CHOC), has made important steps toward streamlining and accelerating this type of research.

To strengthen these efforts, the IOM committee believes that the NCATS-CTSA Steering Committee should identify a relatively small number of CTSAs with established expertise that provide outstanding efforts in child health research as leaders in this arena. This would not preclude other CTSAs from being involved in child health research. Instead, the IOM committee hopes that such focused efforts would encourage and promote collaborations among CTSAs for multisite studies and other efforts. The committee also believes that CTSAs should be engaged in a life-span approach that includes research on the transition from adolescence into adulthood.

As part of a learning health care system, those involved in child health research need to be sure that this area of investigation is well positioned to fully embrace the use of electronic health records for research purposes and to actively partner with practice-based research networks. Implementing these types of strategies will allow researchers to understand what is occurring in clinical practice and will allow pediatric health care providers, patients, and families to learn about new medications, therapeutics, and preventive measures.

Recommendation 7: *Strengthen Clinical and Translational Research Relevant to Child Health*

NCATS should collaborate with the CTSA Consortium Child Health Oversight Committee to strengthen clinical and translational research relevant to child health through efforts to

- **identify and designate CTSAs with expertise in child health research as leaders in advancing clinical and translational research relevant to child health and as coordinators for CTSA programwide efforts and other collaborative efforts in this research; and**
- **promote and increase community engagement specific to child health by**

  o **raising awareness of the opportunities for children and families to participate in research efforts with clear information conveyed on the risks and potential benefits; and**
  o **involving parents, patients, and family members more fully at all stages of the research process, including identifying priorities and setting research agendas.**

CONCLUSION: OPPORTUNITIES FOR ACTION

With the ultimate goal of improving human health, the CTSA Program now has the opportunity to propel clinical and translational research efforts forward rapidly. To move to CTSA 2.0, the CTSA

Program can build on its foundation; draw on the creativity and dedication of CTSA principal investigators, researchers, and staff; use the ever-expanding capabilities of informatics and other technologies; share data and research support tools as openly and freely as possible; and fully engage new cadres of researchers focused on team-based science.

The IOM committee believes that the CTSA Program should be the national leader for advancing innovative and transformative clinical and translational research to improve human health. To achieve this, the CTSA Program should reshape its goals to reflect its new location within NCATS; build on the work of individual CTSAs to provide institutional leadership; focus on team-based education and training; and establish a national network that will accelerate the development of new diagnostics, therapeutics, and preventive interventions and, at the same time, will drive innovation in clinical and translational research methods, processes, tools, and resources. The committee's recommendations are summarized in Box S-1.

Because the CTSA Program is not disease specific in its orientation, strong collaborations must be forged across disciplinary units within individual CTSA institutions and with other NIH institutes and centers, as well as with other government funders, industry, philanthropies, and community organizations. The CTSA Program should continue to lead efforts in expanding and diversifying the research workforce and to coordinate and advance child health research by streamlining and building on the expertise of individual CTSAs. In all these efforts, community engagement is essential.

In short, the contributions of the individual CTSAs and the CTSA Program are vital to the clinical and translational research enterprise, and the nation's health can benefit greatly from strengthening their efforts.

BOX S-1
Overview of Recommendations[a]

The next steps for the Clinical and Translational Science Awards (CTSA) Program and opportunities for advancing clinical and translational research are as follows:

- Strengthen leadership of the CTSA Program by the National Center for Advancing Translational Sciences (NCATS).
- Reconfigure and streamline the CTSA Consortium.
- Build on the strengths of individual CTSAs across the spectrum of clinical and translational research.
- Formalize and standardize evaluation processes for individual CTSAs and the CTSA Program.
- Advance innovation in education and training programs.
- Ensure community engagement in all phases of research.
- Strengthen clinical and translational research relevant to child health.

[a]The full text of the recommendations appears throughout the summary and in Chapters 3 and 4 of the report.

1

Introduction

During the past half-century, biomedical research has expanded exponentially, becoming increasingly complex (IOM, 2013). As a result of improved scientific knowledge, the biomedical research enterprise in the United States has witnessed many successes that offer the promise of improved human health. For example, advances in the fields of genomics and proteomics have led to new targeted diagnostic tools and therapies for diseases as diverse as lung cancer, schizophrenia, and cystic fibrosis (IOM, 2012).

Despite the production of new data and numerous publications disseminating these research findings, translating the results of basic and clinical research into clinical and community practice has been slow and cumbersome, and many years may pass before the benefits of basic science discoveries and clinical investigations reach individual patients and communities. Barriers to translation include long research timelines; the large number of clinical trials that must be abandoned because of limited enrollment; data-sharing challenges; a lack of available resources (including investigators, study participants, and financial support for clinical trials); and increasing costs, complexity, and regulatory burdens (Collins, 2011; Kitterman et al., 2011; NCATS, 2013d; Zerhouni, 2005). These persistent challenges required a new approach to accelerating the translation of research to clinical applications and maximizing improvements in individual and public health.

Recognizing the need for a new research paradigm, the National Institutes of Health (NIH) developed a *Roadmap for Medical Research* in 2004 to focus efforts on the challenges facing medical research (NIH, 2006, 2011, 2013a; Zerhouni, 2005). The NIH Roadmap sought to facilitate new pathways to discovery; promote interdisciplinary and collaborative research teams; and "re-engineer the clinical research enterprise" by harmonizing regulatory policies, encouraging multidisciplinary training, and facilitating the establishment of academic homes for clinical and translational research (NIH, 2006; Zerhouni, 2003).

As part of its effort to implement its Roadmap and spur clinical and translational research, the NIH established the Clinical and Translational Science Awards (CTSA) Program. The CTSA Program was designed to "provide integrated intellectual and physical resources for the conduct of original clinical and translational science" (Zerhouni, 2005, p. 1622), and individual CTSA sites were intended to serve as "catalysts and test beds for policies and practices that can benefit clinical and translational research organizations throughout the country" (Zerhouni, 2006, p. 4). The CTSA Program originally focused on "re-engineering existing capabilities at medical research institutions and developing new resources in the areas of clinical and translational research training, community outreach and informatics" (NCATS, 2013a). Although the CTSA Program does not directly fund or conduct large-scale clinical and translational research, it supports the development and application of shared resources and innovative technologies for clinical and translational studies across the full spectrum of research (NIH, 2012b). Consistent with NIH's Roadmap, the CTSA Program's initial goals were to

- "create academic homes for clinical and translational research;
- provide investigators and research teams with research cores, tools and a local environment that encourages and facilitates the conduct of clinical and translational research, including with community and industry partners; and
- train the scientific workforce needed for the translational sciences" (NCATS, 2013a).

Diverse groups of stakeholders (researchers, funders, the public, and congressional representatives) increasingly seek evidence that the enormous U.S. investment in biomedical research, including the CTSA Program, is bearing tangible fruit in the form of new and better preventive and treatment options. A 2011 congressional conference report highlighted the success and additional promise of the CTSA Program and "urge[d] NIH to support a study by the Institute of Medicine to evaluate the CTSA program and to recommend whether changes to the current mission are needed" (U.S. Congress, 2011). The report specified the charge as follows:

CTSAs now represent an investment of half a decade of innovation in translational research. To ensure the benefits of this investment are maintained, the conferees urge NIH to support a study by the IOM that would evaluate the CTSA program and recommend whether changes to the current mission are needed. The review should include stakeholders' input and be available no later than 18 months after the enactment of this bill. (U.S. Congress, 2011, p. 1137)

SCOPE OF WORK AND STUDY PROCESS

In 2012 the NIH contracted with the Institute of Medicine (IOM) to conduct a consensus study to review the CTSA Program. The IOM convened a 13-member committee with expertise in community outreach and engagement, public health and health policy, bioethics, education and training, pharmaceutical research and development, program evaluation, clinical and biomedical research, and child health research, along the continuum of clinical and translation research (Appendix B).

The committee's statement of task (see Box 1-1) directed it to assess the CTSA Program and its mission and strategic goals and to offer advice on the implementation of the program by the National Center for Advancing Translational Sciences (NCATS), while exploring the contributions of CTSAs in accelerating the development of new therapeutics, facilitating disease-specific research and child health research, and enhancing the integration of research funded by NIH institutes and centers. When presenting the charge to the committee at its first meeting in October 2012, NCATS leaders offered the following questions to help clarify the statement of task:

- "Is the breadth of the program supporting T1 through T4 research appropriate?
- Should the goal of creating an academic home for clinical and translational sciences continue to be a major focus of the CTSA program?
- Are CTSAs effectively providing innovative education, training, and career development support to meet the needs of the biomedical research workforce? How could this aspect of the program be strengthened?

BOX 1-1
Committee to Review the Clinical and Translational
Science Awards Program at the National Center
for Advancing Translation Sciences
Statement of Task

In response to a request from the National Institutes of Health (NIH), the Institute of Medicine (IOM) will assemble an ad hoc expert committee to provide an independent appraisal of and advice on the NIH Clinical and Translational Science Awards (CTSA) Program as it will be implemented by the newly formed National Center for Advancing Translational Sciences (NCATS). The current mission of the CTSA program includes services and infrastructure support for the full continuum of clinical and translational research. The services provided by CTSAs have supported T1 through T4 research, with primary emphasis on support for human subjects research extending from first-in-man and proof-of-concept studies through efficacy and effectiveness studies, and including research on how to achieve community and patient engagement, implementation and dissemination sciences, and behavioral research.

The IOM committee will review existing evaluations and available stakeholder input on the program, and will seek additional stakeholder input as needed. Based on this assessment, the committee will provide recommendations on the appropriateness of the program's current mission and overarching goals and whether changes are needed. This study will explore the contributions of the CTSAs in accelerating the development of new therapeutics with consideration given to the role of the CTSA program in facilitating disease-specific research and pediatric research and in enhancing the integration of programs funded by the categorical NIH Institutes and Centers.

- Are the CTSAs configured effectively to accelerate new therapeutics, and if not, what changes should be implemented?" (Briggs and Austin, 2012).

Throughout this study, the committee considered these questions and used a forward-looking approach to respond to its statement of task. This report builds on previous program evaluations and assessments, although it was not designed to provide a comprehensive and in-depth evaluation of the operations, administration, or achievements of individual CTSA sites or the program as a whole. The committee's advice and recommendations are intended to help NCATS implement the program effectively and enable the full realization of its potential.

During the course of its work, the committee held four meetings, two public workshops, and four open-session conference calls to solicit input about the successes, challenges, and future directions of the CTSA Program (Appendix A). Throughout the study, the committee heard from a number of CTSA principal investigators (PIs) and researchers, members of the NIH and NCATS leadership, community and patient advocacy organizations, industry partners and representatives, and thought leaders and researchers in the clinical and translational sciences arena who were not connected to the CTSA Program. As part of its assessment, the committee reviewed the scientific literature, previous CTSA Program evaluations, available progress reports, responses to formal NIH requests for information (RFIs) related to the CTSA Program, information submitted by a range of CTSA Consortium committees and stakeholder groups, and data and recommendations from other relevant working groups and stakeholder meetings. The committee's work was also informed by responses to a series of public input questions that focused on the CTSA Program's mission and strategic goals and its role in advancing research along the continuum of clinical and translational science.[1]

CLINICAL AND TRANSLATIONAL RESEARCH

Translational research means different things to different people
but it seems important to almost everyone.

—Steven Woolf (Woolf, 2008)

The CTSA Program's focus, by definition, is on clinical and translational research. *Clinical research* involves human participants and includes epidemiological and behavioral studies; outcome and health services research; and patient-oriented research, such as the study of disease pathology and mechanisms, development and testing of therapeutic interventions or technologies, and clinical trials (NIH, 2013b). The NIH's definition of *translational research* includes two broad areas: the translation of basic science and preclinical discoveries into human subject research and the subsequent translation of clinical trial results, research findings, and knowledge into practice in clinical and community settings (NIH, 2013b). For the purposes of this report, however, the committee has adopted a conceptual model of translational research that exists along a dynamic continuum that connects basic research findings to decisions made within clinical settings and interventions that are applied

---

[1]Public testimony and other materials submitted to the committee are available by request through the National Academies' Public Access Records Office.

in community and public health settings to improve health broadly. Figure 1-1 defines and illustrates the conceptual progression across the five phases of translational research, from the initial stages of research (such as preclinical and animal models) to large-scale research in communities and populations. The translational phases along this continuum are sometimes referred to as "bench-to-bedside" and "bedside-to-community" (Blumberg et al., 2012; ITHS, 2013; Khoury et al., 2007).

Despite efforts to raise the profile and improve the accessibility of translational research, misconceptions persist about its scope, and many people conflate the concepts of clinical and translational research. As illustrated below, the continuum of translational research (T0–T4) is broader than clinical research (T1–T3). Although the depiction of the separate phases of translational research above suggests a linear model with a finite beginning and end, in reality the operational phases of translational research include many feedback loops. Its process is more circular and interdependent across research phases, requiring continuous data gathering, analysis, dissemination, and interaction (see Figure 1-2). In formation sharing at each stage ensures that researchers are meeting patient and community health needs and that progress in the clinic and

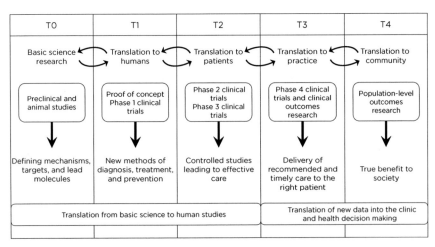

FIGURE 1-1 Operational phases of translational research (T0–T4).
SOURCE: Adapted with permission from Macmillan Publishers Ltd.: *Nature Medicine* (Blumberg et al., 2012), copyright 2012.

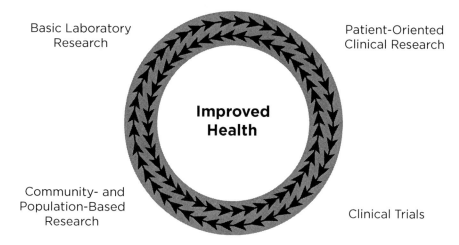

Basic Laboratory Research

Patient-Oriented Clinical Research

Improved Health

Community- and Population-Based Research

Clinical Trials

FIGURE 1-2 An integrated model of clinical and translational research. SOURCE: Adapted from Austin, 2013.

community, in turn, informs the work in the laboratory. As a result, the impact of translational research on health improvements hinges on an integrated and responsive research infrastructure, similar to models of a "learning health care system" (discussed in Chapter 2).

The value of continuous feedback from communities to researchers is illustrated by three of the many advances in clinical and translational research the CTSA Program has achieved (see Box 1-2), which are being used by individuals and communities to improve health and quality of life.

BOX 1-2
Examples of Advances Accomplished Through Successful Clinical and Translational Research

Cystic fibrosis. On January 31, 2012, the Food and Drug Administration (FDA) approved the drug Kalydeco for people with a rare form of cystic fibrosis. Kalydeco is the first drug to target the underlying cause of this type of cystic fibrosis and is the result of a unique collaboration between the Cystic Fibrosis Foundation, Vertex Pharmaceuticals, and 10 CTSA institutions. This collaboration facilitated clinical trials that garnered FDA approval (FDA, 2012; NCATS, 2012, 2013b).

Diabetes. To improve the health of individuals with diabetes or those who are at risk of developing diabetes, investigators at CTSAs in California, Connecticut, and South Carolina are working with local communities to explore models of diabetes prevention and interventions tailored to the needs of those communities. For example, researchers at Yale University are currently testing and implementing a 12-week intervention at a local community health center that features intensive lifestyle changes for women with pre-diabetes (NIH, 2012b; Tamborlane, 2009; Yale School of Medicine, 2012a,b).

OVERVIEW OF THE CTSA PROGRAM

History

The CTSA Program is a direct outgrowth of the NIH's General Clinical Research Center (GCRC) Program, which for more than 40 years provided clinical research infrastructure funding.[2] The GCRCs provided clinical researchers with dedicated inpatient beds, outpatient units, core laboratory support, and staffing support (e.g., research nurses, laboratory technicians, biostatisticians) (Robertson and Tung, 2001). Beginning in 2005, with the implementation of the NIH Roadmap and NIH's efforts to revitalize its work in clinical and translational research, the GCRC Program was phased out. Funding from that program was redirected and consolidated with other existing resources (e.g., T- and K-training and career development awards), along with additional support from the NIH Common Fund, to launch the CTSA Program (NIH, 2005; Shurin, 2008).

In 2006, 12 CTSA sites were funded through 5-year cooperative agreements as a first step toward establishing academic homes for clinical and translational research (Briggs and Austin, 2012; NIH, 2005; OIG, 2011). Institutional CTSA funding levels were based on the applicant's previous GCRC funding and other NIH training awards (Briggs and Austin, 2012). A number of GCRC institutions applied for and received CTSA Program funding, and their GCRC clinical research units and associated resources were folded into the new program (NIH, 2012a). Following the first round of awards, the NIH added 5 to 14 new CTSA sites annually until, by the end of 2012, the program reached capacity at 61

---

[2]The GCRCs began in the early 1960s and focused on metabolic and nutritional studies (Briggs and Austin, 2012; Robertson and Tung, 2001). Researchers applied to the GCRC in a specific institution to use its clinical research units for their institutional review board (IRB)-approved research. In 2005 there were 78 GCRC sites with a total budget of approximately $288 million (Briggs and Austin, 2012).

sites nationwide (see Figure 1-3) (Briggs and Austin, 2012; Reis et al., 2010). The annual budgets for these sites range from $4 million to $23 million (Briggs and Austin, 2012; CTSA Central, 2013a), and the total annual budget for the program for fiscal year (FY) 2012 was $461 million.

The CTSA Program was administered by the National Center for Research Resources (NCRR) through 2011, when the Consolidated Appropriations Act of 2012 (Public Law 112-74) established NCATS and dissolved the NCRR (Collins, 2011; Reed et al., 2012). The NCATS mission focuses on catalyzing innovative methods and technologies related to the development of diagnostics and therapeutics, and it became home to the CTSA Program and several smaller, related NIH programs. The CTSA Program accounted for approximately 80 percent of the NCATS budget in FY2012 (Briggs and Austin, 2012).

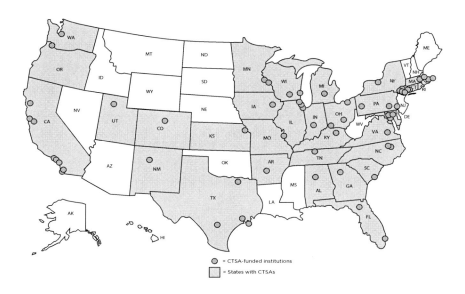

FIGURE 1-3 CTSA-funded institutions and participating states.
SOURCE: CTSA Central, 2013a. Reprinted with permission from the National Institutes of Health, U.S. Department of Health and Human Services.

During the initial transition period and under interim leadership, NCATS sought input from a wide range of stakeholders through a variety of mechanisms (e.g., RFIs, internal NIH working groups) on the implementation of the CTSA Program and strategies for enhancing it. As NCATS begins to lead the program forward, it is taking incremental steps to reshape its work. For example, its first request for applications (RFA) signaled more flexibility in focus for individual CTSAs (see Chapter 3) and a new funding structure in which support for individual CTSAs will be based on their institution's total NIH research funding base (NIH, 2012c).

Structure of the CTSA Program

Today's CTSA Program facilitates the training and education of investigators and fosters a collaborative environment to promote improvements in the quality, safety, efficiency, and cost-effectiveness of clinical and translational research. It does not focus on any one disease or disorder, although individual CTSA sites and projects may do so (NIH, 2012c). The program has a complex, multilevel organizational and oversight structure involving individual institutions, the CTSA Consortium, the CTSA Coordinating Center, and NCATS. NCATS's Division of Clinical Innovation oversees the CTSA Program and provides funding and other resource support for individual CTSA sites.

Individual CTSAs

At the heart of the CTSA Program are the 61 individual CTSAs established in academic health centers and other institutions across the United States and the commitment and ingenuity of the researchers and partners who work with them. These institutions have some flexibility in how to structure their individual programs. Many CTSAs are housed in medical schools and collaborate with other departments and schools in their universities, as well as with other universities, hospitals, and health care systems (CTSA Central, 2013h). Each CTSA must set up an external advisory committee that meets annually to provide advice on structure, progress, and challenges of the program (NIH, 2012c). Many CTSAs also have established internal advisory committees and other advisory and governance committees (e.g., executive committees, community advisory boards).

Because CTSA funding levels vary widely across sites, the scope of their activities also varies (see also Chapter 3). In general, CTSA sites provide an array of training and research resources and support tools designed to help investigators conduct promising research, including

- *core facilities* (e.g., translational technologies, core laboratory services, and novel methodologies, such as specific embryonic stem cell lines, nanotechnology, and epigenomics);
- *biomedical informatics* (e.g., behavioral data analysis, geographic coding, proteomics, registration for trials through tools such as ResearchMatch [see Chapter 3], customized software);
- *pilot funding* (e.g., through CTSA pilots, institutional pilots, trainee and scholar pilot programs, and partnerships with industry and not-for-profit organizations);
- *regulatory knowledge and support* (e.g., auditing and compliance measures, HIPAA compliance, conflicts-of-interest management, protocol development and preparation, and IRB agreements);
- *biostatistics, epidemiology, research design, and ethics* (e.g., ethics consultations, adaptive trial design, randomization and blinding, statistical modeling and analysis, multicenter coordination, grant application support);
- *participant and clinical interaction resources* (e.g., cost recovery planning, case report form development and reporting compliance, research nurse support, research subject advocacy); and
- *community engagement efforts and resources* (e.g., adult literacy assessment, cultural competency training, public databases, promotion of research participation) (Rosenblum, 2012).

CTSA Consortium Committees and Coordinating Center

CTSA Consortium committees From the outset of the program, the NIH charged the CTSAs with developing a national consortium to promote the identification and use of best research practices (Berglund and Tarantal, 2009). The original funding announcement called for a consortium steering committee comprised of CTSA PIs. In addition, it directed that subcommittees be formed around NIH-identified key functions (e.g., education, informatics, regulation) (NIH, 2005). Further details on the governance and structure of the CTSA Consortium and its committees were formalized in 2008 as part of the PI-directed strategic planning process. At that time, the CTSA Program consisted of two dozen individual

CTSAs (Reis et al., 2010). The initial NIH guidance and the strategic planning effort formed the basis for the complex, multi-tiered CTSA Consortium committee structure that exists today, which includes hundreds of participants.

The CTSAs' collaborative efforts are overseen by three leadership committees:

- The *Consortium Executive Committee* is the main governing body and has 31 members (more than 20 of whom are voting members), including leadership of the Consortium Steering Committee (described below), 5 CTSA PIs, NCATS staff, and other members who serve 1-year terms. Its purpose, in part, is to facilitate interactions among the PIs, NCATS staff, and the various consortium committees (CTSA Central, 2013e).

- The *Consortium Steering Committee* has more than 175 members (more than 85 of whom at voting members), including PIs from each CTSA institution and representatives from NCATS and a number of other NIH institutes and centers. It provides leadership and management of the consortium and is responsible for setting strategic goals and priorities (CTSA Central, 2013g).

- The *CTSA Consortium Child Health Oversight Committee* focuses on overcoming barriers and promoting opportunities for child health research and has more than 230 members, almost 60 of whom are voting members (also discussed in Chapter 4).

In addition to the leadership committees, CTSA PIs, researchers, and staff coordinate collaborative efforts and work to improve program functioning through numerous CTSA Consortium committees, interest groups, working groups, and task forces that have evolved with the growth of the program (see Box 1-3). Five strategic goal committees consist of 20 to 30 members each. These committees identify and prioritize efforts related to achieving the strategic goals defined in 2008 (CTSA Central, 2013b; Reis et al., 2010).

Fourteen key function committees discuss crosscutting issues, promote collaboration, and identify and implement best practices. The key function committees reflect areas deemed essential to the program's mission, and some of them have been required in NIH funding announcements. The number and focus of the key function committees have fluctuated over the life of the CTSA program as priorities shifted (Evanoff, 2012). Many of these committees include more than 100 members and have subcommittees, working groups, and task forces (CTSA Central, 2013c). In addition, numerous informal groups of CTSA researchers have developed around topics of mutual interest.

After the development of the strategic goals in 2008, an effort was made to map the key functions to correspond to one or more of program strategic goals (Reis et al., 2010). Table 1-1 indicates that, although related, strategic goals and key function groups do not consistently align. A commitment to participate in CTSA Consortium efforts, including the committees, has been a condition of receiving a CTSA award (NIH, 2010). All the committees described above convene regular conference calls to discuss progress and share best practices. The committees comprise PIs and researchers who take on these extra responsibilities in addition to their work at their institution's CTSA.

BOX 1-3
CTSA Consortium Committees and Working Groups

Consortium Leadership Committee

- Consortium Executive Committee
- Consortium Steering Committee
- CTSA Consortium Child Health Oversight Committee

Consortium Strategic Goal Committees

- Strategic Goal Committee 1–National Clinical and Translational Research Capability
- Strategic Goal Committee 2–Training and Career Development of Clinical/Translational Scientists
- Strategic Goal Committee 3–Enhancing Consortium-Wide Collaborations
- Strategic Goal Committee 4–Enhancing the Health of Our Communities and the Nation
- Strategic Goal Committee 5–T1 Translational Research

Key Function Committees

- Administration Key Function Committee
- Biostatistics/Epidemiology/Research Design Key Function Committee
- Clinical Research Ethics Key Function Committee
- Clinical Research Management Key Function Committee
- Clinical Services Core Key Function Committee
- Communications Key Function Committee
- Community Engagement Key Function Committee

- Comparative Effectiveness Research Key Function Committee
- Education and Career Development Key Function Committee
- Evaluation Key Function Committee
- Informatics Key Function Committee
- Public–Private Partnerships Key Function Committee
- Regulatory Knowledge Key Function Committee
- Translational Key Function Committee

CTSA Thematic Special Interest Groups

- CTSA Nurse Scientist
- CTSA Pain Research Interest Group
- CTSA TEAM (TElemed, teleheAlth, Mhealth)
- CTSA-USCIITG Critical Care Interest Group
- Dentistry and Oral Health
- Emergency Care Researchers
- Neuroscience Researchers
- Sleep Research Network
- VA Research Collaboration
- Women in Clinical and Translational Research Interest Group

SOURCES: CTSA Central, 2013c,f,i.

TABLE 1-1 Alignment of the CTSA Key Function Committees and Strategic Goal Committees

Strategic Goal Committees	1	2	3	4	5
Key Function Committees That Support Strategic Goal Committees					
Clinical Research Management	• X				
Clinical Services Core	• X			•	
Regulatory Knowledge	• X				
Education and Career Development		• X		•	•
Community Engagement				• X	
Comparative Effectiveness Research				• X	
Public–Private Partnerships			•	•	• X
Translational					• X
Communications			• X	•	•
Crosscutting Key Function Committees					
Informatics	•	•	•	•	•
Evaluation	•	•	•	•	•
Biostatistics/Epidemiology/Design	•	•	•	•	•
Clinical Research Ethics	•	•	•	•	•

Strategic Goal Committees	1	2	3	4	5
General Grant/Consortium Operations					
Administration	•	•	•	•	•

NOTE: • = alignment for related agenda topics and deliverable support; X = alignment for reporting purposes and on-going management of deliverables.
SOURCE: https://www.ctsacentral.org/committees (accessed May 6, 2013).

CTSA Consortium Coordinating Center In November 2011, the CTSA Consortium Coordinating Center was established through a competitive application process, which awarded Vanderbilt University a budget of $20 million over 5 years to

- establish a high visibility and accessible "national home" for the CTSA Program;
- manage meetings, projects, and communications of the CTSA Consortium;
- compile and organize the CTSA Consortium's networking resources; and
- develop and disseminate research tools and resources that support translational research (CTSA Central, 2013d; Snyder, 2011).

Since its inception, the coordinating center has taken many steps to standardize and coordinate consortium activities (e.g., project and meeting support, listservs). In its efforts, the coordinating center also attempts to ensure the dissemination of best practices, facilitate the uptake of available tools and resources, and promote collaboration, in part, through its website, CTSACentral.org. The coordinating center facilitated PI efforts to produce a joint publication on the program's transition to NCATS and a joint response to an NCATS RFI regarding opportunities to enhance the CTSA Program (Bernard, 2012; CTSA PIs, 2012; Pulley, 2013). The coordinating center is also striving to improve connections between the CTSA Program and NIH institutes and centers through a new liaison effort. Under that initiative, 40 CTSA PIs are working with 18 NIH institutes and centers to increase communication, awareness of available CTSA resources, and the integration of trans-NIH resources (Bernard, 2012).

ORGANIZATION OF THE REPORT

This report provides the IOM committee's findings and recommendations regarding the progress and potential of NIH's CTSA Program. The report covers the breadth of the statement of task and highlights opportunities to bolster the program and ensure its continued success and sustainability in supporting clinical and translational researchers and serving the needs of the communities CTSAs are linked to and in which they reside. Chapter 2 discusses the ecosystem in which NCATS and the CTSA Program operate and provides the committee's vision for the next phase of the CTSA Program. Chapter 3 emphasizes the need for strong and active leadership by NCATS in establishing a clear vision and mission for the program along with measurable goals; supporting individual CTSAs; partnering and collaborating within the NIH and with external partners; and evaluating and communicating the program's value. Chapter 4 highlights specific opportunities and priorities in the areas of training and education, community engagement, and research related to child health. On the basis of discussions, conclusions, and recommendations outlined in the preceding chapters, in Chapter 5 the report concludes with next steps and potential future directions.

REFERENCES

Austin, C. P. 2013. *National Center for Advancing Translational Sciences: Catalyzing translational innovation.* PowerPoint presented at Meeting 3: IOM Committee to Review the CTSA Program at NCATS, Washington, DC, January 24. http://www.iom.edu/~/media/Files/Activity%20Files/Research/CTSAReview/2013-JAN-24/Chris%20Austin.pdf (accessed February 13, 2013).

Berglund, L., and A. Tarantal. 2009. Strategies for innovation and interdisciplinary translational research: Removal of barriers through the CTSA mechanism. *Journal of Investigative Medicine* 57(2):474–476.

Bernard, G. 2012. *CTSA Consortium Coordinating Center (C4).* PowerPoint presented at Meeting 2: IOM Committee to Review the CTSA Program at NCATS, Washington, DC, December 12. http://www.iom.edu/~/media/Files/Activity%20Files/Research/CTSAReview/2012-DEC-12/3-1%20Gordon%20Bernard.pdf (accessed March 28, 2013).

Blumberg, R. S., B. Dittel, D. Hafler, M. von Herrath, and F. O. Nestle. 2012. Unraveling the autoimmune translational research process layer by layer. *Nature Medicine* 18(1):35–41.

Briggs, J., and C. P. Austin. 2012. *NCATS and the evolution of the Clinical and Translational Science Awards (CTSA) Program.* PowerPoint presented at Meeting 1: IOM Committee to Review the CTSA Program at NCATS, Washington, DC, October 29. http://www.iom.edu/~/media/Files/activity%20Files/Research/CTSAReview/2012-OCT-29/IOM%20Briggs-Austin%20102912.pdf (accessed February 13, 2013).

Collins, F. S. 2011. Reengineering translational science: The time is right. *Science Translational Medicine* 3(90):1–6.

CTSA (Clinical and Translational Science Awards) Central. 2013a. *About the CTSA Consortium.* https://www.ctsacentral.org/about-us/ctsa (accessed February 13, 2013).

———. 2013b. *Clinical and Translational Science Awards.* https://www.ctsacentral.org (accessed March 26, 2013).

———. 2013c. *Consortium committees.* https://www.ctsacentral.org/committees (accessed February 13, 2013).

———. 2013d. *CTSA Consortium Coordinating Center (C4).* https://www.ctsacentral.org/about-us/c4 (accessed February 13, 2013).

———. 2013e. *CTSA Consortium Executive Committee.* https://www.ctsacentral.org/committee/ctsa-consortium-executive-committee (accessed February 13, 2013).

———. 2013f. *CTSA Consortium leadership.* https://www.ctsacentral.org/consortium/leadership (accessed April 18, 2013, 2013).

———. 2013g. *CTSA Consortium Steering Committee.* https://www.ctsacentral.org/committee/ctsa-consortium-steering-committee (accessed February 13, 2013).

———. 2013h. *CTSA institutions.* https://www.ctsacentral.org/institutions (accessed February 13, 2013).

———. 2013i. *Thematic special interest groups.* https://www.ctsacentral.org/tsig (accessed April 1, 2013).

CTSA PIs (Principal Investigators). 2012. Preparedness of the CTSA's structural and scientific assets to support the mission of the National Center for Advancing Translational Sciences (NCATS). *Clinical and Translational Science* 5(2):121–129.

Evanoff, B. 2012. *CTSA Consortium governance and organization.* PowerPoint presented at Meeting 1: IOM Committee to Review the CTSA Program at NCATS, Washington, DC, October 29. http://www.iom.edu/~/media/Files/Activity%20Files/Research/CTSAReview/2012-OCT-29/CTSA%20presentations/1-Evanoff%20IOM%20committee.pdf (accessed March 28, 2013).

FDA (Food and Drug Administration). 2012. *FDA approves Kalydeco to treat rare form of cystic fibrosis.* http://www.fda.gov/NewsEvents/Newsroom/PressAnnouncements/ucm289633.htm (accessed February 13, 2013).

IOM (Institute of Medicine). 2012. *Genome-based therapeutics: Targeted drug discovery and development: Workshop summary.* Washington, DC: The National Academies Press.

―――. 2013. *Best care at lower cost: The path to continuously learning health care in America.* Washington, DC: The National Academies Press.

ITHS (Institute of Translational Health Sciences). 2013. *Translational research: T-phases of translational health research.* https://www.iths.org/about/translational (accessed February 13, 2013).

Khoury, M. J., M. Gwinn, P. W. Yoon, N. Dowling, C. A. Moore, and L. Bradley. 2007. The continuum of translation research in genomic medicine: How can we accelerate the appropriate integration of human genome discoveries into health care and disease prevention? *Genetics in Medicine* 9(10):665–674.

Kitterman, D. R., S. K. Cheng, D. M. Dilts, and E. S. Orwoll. 2011. The prevalence and economic impact of low-enrolling clinical studies at an academic medical center. *Academic Medicine* 86(11):1360–1366.

NCATS (National Center for Advancing Translational Sciences). 2012. *Clinical and Translational Awards factsheet.* http://www.ncats.nih.gov/files/ctsa-factsheet.pdf (accessed March 26, 2013).

―――. 2013a. *About the CTSA Program.* http://www.ncats.nih.gov/research/cts/ctsa/about/about.html (accessed April 8, 2013).

―――. 2013b. *New drug for rare type of cystic fibrosis.* http://www.ncats.nih.gov/news-and-events/features/cystic-fibrosis.html (accessed April 8, 2013).

―――. 2013c. *Pitt researchers work to restore function in paralysis patients.* http://www.ncats.nih.gov/news-and-events/features/brain-comp.html (accessed April 8, 2013).

―――. 2013d. *Research: Clinical and translational science.* http://www.ncats.nih.gov/research/cts/cts.html (accessed April 8, 2013).

NIH (National Institutes of Health). 2005. *RFA-RM-06-002: Institutional Clinical and Translational Science Award (U54).* http://grants.nih.gov/grants/guide/rfa-files/RFA-RM-06-002.html (accessed February 13, 2013).

―――. 2006. *NIH roadmap for medical research fact sheet.* http://opasi.nih.gov/documents/NIHRoadmap_FactSheet_Aug06.pdf (accessed February 13, 2013).

―――. 2010. *RFA-RM-10-001: Institutional Clinical and Translational Science Award (U54).* http://grants.nih.gov/grants/guide/rfa-files/RFA-RM-10-001.html (accessed March 28, 2013).

―――. 2011. *Programs: About the NIH roadmap.* http://commonfund.nih.gov/aboutroadmap.aspx (accessed March 26, 2013).

―――. 2012a. *National Center for Research Resources: Major extramural programs.* http://www.nih.gov/about/almanac/organization/NCRR.htm#programs (accessed April 26, 2013).

―――. 2012b. *Progress report 2009–2011 Clinical and Translational Science Awards: Foundations for accelerated discovery and efficient translation.* http://www.ncats.nih.gov/ctsa_2011 (accessed March 26, 2013).

————. 2012c. *RFA-TR-12-006: Institutional Clinical and Translational Science Award (U54).* http://grants.nih.gov/grants/guide/rfa-files/rfa-tr-12-006.html (accessed February 13, 2013).

————. 2013a. *About NIH.* http://www.nih.gov/about (accessed February 13, 2013).

————. 2013b. *Glossary and acronym list.* http://grants.nih.gov/grants/glossary.htm (accessed February 13. 2013).

OIG (Office of the Inspector General). 2011. *NIH administration of the Clinical and Translational Science Awards Program.* https://oig.hhs.gov/oei/reports/oei-07-09-00300.pdf (accessed April 8, 2013).

Pulley, J. 2013. *CTSA PI response to RFI NOT-TR-12-003.* Submitted to the IOM Committee on January 6. Available by request through the National Academies' Public Access Records Office.

Reed, J. C., E. L. White, J. Aube, C. Lindsley, M. Li, L. Sklar, and S. Schreiber. 2012. The NIH's role in accelerating translational sciences. *Nature Biotechnology* 30(1):16–19.

Reis, S. E., L. Berglund, G. R. Bernard, R. M. Califf, G. A. FitzGerald, and P. C. Johnson. 2010. Reengineering the national clinical and translational research enterprise: The strategic plan of the National Clinical and Translational Science Awards Consortium. *Academic Medicine* 85(3):463–469.

Robertson, D., and C.-S. Tung. 2001. Linking molecular and bedside research: Designing a clinical research infrastructure. *Journal of Molecular Medicine* 79(12):686–694.

Rosenblum, D. 2012. Access to core facilities and other research resources provided by the Clinical and Translational Science Awards. *Clinical and Translational Science* 5(1):78–82.

Shurin, S. B. 2008. Clinical Translational Science Awards: Opportunities and challenges. *Clinical and Translational Science* 1(1):4.

Snyder, B. 2011. VUMC to lead national CTSA consortium. *Reporter: Vanderbilt University Medical Center's Weekly Newspaper.* http://www.mc.vanderbilt.edu/reporter/index.html?ID=10883 (accessed February 13, 2013).

Tamborlane, W. 2009. *Changing lifestyles for better health: Diabetes mellitus behavioral intensive lifestyle intervention, NCT00848757.* http://clinicaltrials.gov/show/nct00848757 (accessed February 13, 2013).

U.S. Congress, House of Representatives. 2011. *Military Constructions and Veterans Affairs and Related Agencies Appropriations Act: Conference report to accompany HR 2055*, 112th Cong., 1st sess. http://www.gpo.gov/fdsys/pkg/CRPT-112hrpt331/pdf/CRPT-112hrpt331.pdf (accessed May 6, 2013).

Woolf, S. H. 2008. The meaning of translational research and why it matters. *JAMA* 299(2):211–213.

Yale School of Medicine. 2012a. *Diabetes Endocrinology Research Center: Clinical trials.* http://derc.yale.edu/cores/translational/clinicaltrials/index. aspx (accessed February 13, 2013).

————. 2012b. *Diabetes Endocrinology Research Center: Diabetes translational core.* http://derc.yale.edu/cores/translational/index.aspx (accessed February 13, 2013).

Zerhouni, E. A. 2003. The NIH Roadmap. *Science* 302(5642):63–72.

————. 2005. Translational and clinical science—time for a new vision. *New England Journal of Medicine* 353(15):1621–1623.

————. 2006. Clinical and Translational Science Awards: A framework for a national research agenda. *Translational Research* 148(1):4–5.

2

A Vision for the CTSA Program in a Changing Landscape

The Clinical and Translational Science Awards (CTSA) Program does not exist in isolation; it is part of a larger clinical and translational research ecosystem that plays a vital role in an increasingly complex and dynamic U.S. health care system. The individual CTSAs were originally designed as a set of academic focal points (or academic "homes") for facilitating clinical and translational research. To better determine whether the CTSA Program's mission and goals remain appropriate, as requested in its statement of task, the Institute of Medicine (IOM) committee examined how the changing U.S. health care landscape affects the relationship between the CTSA Program and the larger clinical and translational research ecosystem.

This chapter begins by exploring some of these large-scale changes and their impact on clinical and translational research and concludes by describing a new vision for the CTSA Program and opportunities for the National Center for Advancing Translational Sciences (NCATS) to fulfill this vision.

THE CURRENT U.S. HEALTH CARE RESEARCH LANDSCAPE

Decades of innovation and technological advances have led to progress in biomedical sciences, medicine, and public health, contributing to increased life expectancy and improved individual and population health. National initiatives and an emphasis on public reporting of quality measures have improved some specific health outcomes and the management of chronic diseases (Commonwealth Fund, 2011). For example, in recent decades there have been strides in controlling high blood pressure and in improving factors associated with diabetes control (i.e., A1C, blood pressure, and cholesterol) (Casagrande et al., 2013; Commonwealth Fund, 2011). Another significant change is that medical screening and diagnostics continue to move to less expensive settings—from hospitals, to physician offices, to retail clinics, to homes. For example, rapid advances in screening tools led the Food and Drug Administration (FDA) to approve the first in-home testing kit for HIV in 2012 (Chappel et al., 2009; FDA, 2012). At the same time, sophisticated laboratory techniques, combined with a growing data infrastructure and new analytic tools, are reshaping research. For example, researchers and entrepreneurs now have online access to an ever-expanding library of human genome sequence data generated by the 1000 Genomes Project, provided at no cost through the Amazon Web Services cloud (EMBL-EBI, 2013; NIH, 2012a).

The accelerating pace of scientific discoveries has a downside as well. The complexity of the U.S. health care system has increased, contributing to inconsistent health care quality, escalating costs, inequities in access, and shortcomings in improvement in population health outcomes (IOM, 2013a). The IOM has reported that systematic underuse, misuse, and overuse of medical treatments significantly and negatively affect the overall quality and safety of health care and put individual patients at risk (IOM, 1998, 2001, 2013a). In response to these persistent challenges, diverse stakeholders (e.g., policy makers, payers, health care professionals, researchers, industry representatives, community advocacy groups, and individual patients) have called for dramatic changes in health care research and delivery. Efforts are under way to increase accountability for the effectiveness and efficiency of the U.S. health care system by aligning stakeholder interests around the concept of value (Public Law 111-148) (Porter, 2010; Porter and Teisberg, 2006). Across the United States, momentum is growing in support of a learning health care system that promotes novel partnerships and collaborations around research networks and clinical and delivery system innovations to continually improve health care value.

A learning health care system is founded on the concept of continuous improvement and the imperative to translate "what we know" into "what we do." Such a system fuels greater value in health care by harnessing the promise of new technological capabilities, market opportunities, and policies across the health care landscape (IOM, 2013a). Leaders in the public and private sectors are generating and using real-time knowledge to improve outcomes; engaging patients, families, and communities in decisions related to health and health care; and promoting a new culture of care committed to sustained improvement in human health and health care efficiency (IOM, 2013a).

Clinical and translational research are integral to a learning health care system, which relies on an "iterative innovation process designed to generate and apply the best evidence for the collaborative health care choices of each patient and provider; to drive the process of discovery as a natural outgrowth of patient care; and to ensure innovation, quality, safety, and value in health care" (Kemp, 2012, p. 1).

As Figure 2-1 illustrates, the interconnected forces of clinical research and practice fuel a learning health care system. Researchers and health care providers design and implement care, evaluations, or research based on needs of specific communities and populations, which are identified through needs assessments (external scans) or on the basis of observations of researchers and health care providers (internal scans). The resulting data and analyses measure the effectiveness of particular health care goods, services, and processes. These findings are disseminated to inform clinical practice and research models to improve health. This cyclical relationship allows a learning health care system to stay relevant in an ever-changing health care landscape.

The concepts of a learning health care system and translational research both rely on successful integration of clinical research and practice, which has significant implications for conventional notions of bioethics. The traditional paradigm draws a "sharp distinction between clinical research and practice" (Faden et al., 2013, p. s16). Human subject research, unlike clinical practice, is subject to strict federal regulations that protect research participants,[1] and overall health care system improvement activities must act accordingly (Faden et al., 2013). Regulatory oversight burdens can threaten the health of patients and populations by delaying or obstructing potentially beneficial changes to clinical practice (Millum and Menikoff, 2010), especially if concerns about research oversight limit research utility, analytic rigor, or dissemination of quality improvement data (Faden et al., 2013).

CTSAs can play a crucial role in recalibrating the longtime ethical divide between research and clinical care. The Ethics Consultation

---

[1]See, for example, 45 C.F.R. 46.

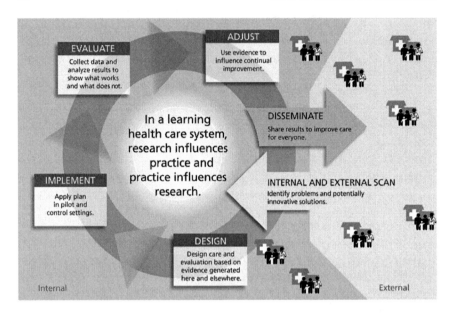

FIGURE 2-1 The learning health care system.
SOURCE: Larson et al., 2013. Reprinted with permission from Radcliffe Publishing.

Working Group, which includes members from 40 CTSAs, "creat[es] a professional community to share strategies, policies, practices, approaches, and information" on this topic (NCATS, 2012, p. 20). By serving as best-practices laboratories in this new ethics environment and by disseminating lessons learned, CTSAs have the potential to advance a new regulatory framework in which the interests in improving health care for patients and protecting individual research participants converge. In addition to the CTSAs' efforts in advancing this new regulatory framework, ongoing collaboration with key research and regulatory agencies, such as the FDA, the National Institutes of Health (NIH), and the Department of Health and Human Services' (HHS's) Office for Human Research Protections, will be necessary.

AN EVOLVING CLINICAL AND TRANSLATIONAL RESEARCH ECOSYSTEM

The clinical and translational research ecosystem currently involves researchers, funders, health care systems, research networks, health professionals, regulators, industry, community stakeholders, and individuals working in varied settings—laboratories, hospitals, academic health centers, community clinics, private practices, and other places patients receive care. The CTSA Program facilitates interactions between stakeholders within the ecosystem and across settings to accelerate progress in clinical and translational research.

The diversity of stakeholders' interests makes the research ecosystem susceptible to a wide range of transformative forces. In the 1970s, for example, clinical and basic research began to diverge; basic biomedical research developed as a distinct discipline, with a separate training and career trajectory (Butler, 2008), a divide that translational research is now trying to address.

Other broader social concerns also affect researchers. With the proliferation of health information systems and technologies, including the use of electronic health records (EHRs) and databases, concerns about individual privacy and the security of health information have intensified, especially around data not directly relevant to health care goods and services (IOM, 2010). Major shifts toward enhanced patient confidentiality (e.g., the Health Insurance Portability and Accountability Act of 1996) have led to greater protection of personal information, but also present challenges in the conduct of efficient and clinical and translational research by "restrict[ing] the manner in which health care providers may use and disclose health information for health research" (Pritts, 2008). These challenges will likely increase as research expands within the context of the learning health care system, with traditional distinctions between clinical care and research blurring and with the role of research participant protections requiring new analysis, clarification, or even revision.

Although advances in biomedical sciences and informatics have vastly expanded opportunities for research, a number of persistent data challenges will need to be overcome in order to realize the full potential of clinical and translational science. For example, interoperability and connectivity issues among data sources, along with privacy concerns, cultural barriers, and lack of incentives, impede data sharing among researchers and across sectors (e.g., academia, industry). Nevertheless, a recent IOM workshop report noted that "research advances derived from data pooling and analysis could improve public health, enhance patient safety, and spur drug development" (IOM, 2013c, p. 1). Fragmentation, lack of standardization/heterogeneity, and the uneven accuracy and quality of available health data are additional challenges for researchers (IOM, 2010, 2013c).

Finally, funding limits are forcing stakeholders to set priorities, share resources, and target their investments. Today, industry's focus has shifted away from the full range of bench-to-bedside discoveries toward investments in potential products that have already completed the early phases of research (Butler, 2008; Reed et al., 2012). Resource scarcity has focused attention on research value, and increasingly stakeholders, including research funders, the public, and Congress, are demanding evidence of returns on investments and greater accountability (Austin, 2013; Reed et al., 2012; Shuster, 2012).

Although "measuring the outcomes of translational research is notoriously difficult" (Butler, 2008, p. 842) for many reasons (e.g., significant time lapses between original clinical trials and measurable impacts on population health or clinical practice), tracking research outcomes is necessary in order to improve accountability and efficiency of translational research, as well as overall health care system performance.

Responding to a Changing Ecosystem

In response to this shifting health care landscape, the clinical and translational research ecosystem has begun to reinvent and realign itself. These adaptations include enhanced collaboration, emerging data and technology, streamlined institutional review board (IRB) processes and enhanced patient protections, broader research participant recruitment efforts, and development of a dynamic research workforce.

Enhanced Collaboration

A growing number of private and public institutions are collaborating to share limited resources for clinical and translational research activities. The resulting coordination is creating broader research networks, enhancing facilitation of investigator-initiated projects, and improving the validity of patient-centered research outcomes.[2] It also has

---

[2]For example, the NIH initiative PROMIS (Patient Reported Outcomes Measurement Information System) was designed to provide flexible yet valid, precise, and responsive assessment tools to measure self-reported health status (Fries et al., 2011; NIH PROMIS, 2013).

the potential to accelerate the translation of research findings into clinical practice (Lieu et al., 2011; Main et al., 2012; Marantz et al., 2011; Melese et al., 2009). These partnerships build on the strength of the stakeholders, expand the stakeholders' reach and capacity, and push boundaries on roles in translational science.

Diverse collaborations and novel roles and partnerships among academic, industry, and nonprofit organizations are emerging. Pfizer's Centers for Therapeutic Innovations are partnering with academic institutions through jointly staffed laboratories and shared access to compound libraries and screening technologies (Pfizer, 2013). Disease advocacy organizations have spun off drug discovery and development entities (e.g., Cystic Fibrosis Foundation Therapeutics, Inc.) (CFF, 2013).

Academic health centers, which once served as the exclusive "home" for clinical investigation, now share the field with other types of research organizations. Health maintenance organizations (HMOs), hospital networks, health care systems, community health centers, and practice-based research networks (PBRNs) have established their own research networks to conduct and facilitate clinical studies (Calmbach et al., 2012; Lieu et al., 2011). The conduct of translational research in primary care settings can lead to improvements in patient care by directly evaluating the feasibility of an intervention or protocol (Calmbach et al., 2012; Fulda et al., 2011). For example, the North Texas Primary Care Practice-Based Research Network (NorTex), housed within the Primary Care Research Center at the University of North Texas Health Science Center, is engaged in a range of studies involving more than 300 physicians at 135 clinics (Fulda et al., 2011). CTSAs provide an opportunity to further strengthen collaborative programs with HMOs and PBRNs in order to accelerate patient-focused research initiatives (also see Chapter 3). The NIH has established the Common Fund's Health Care Systems (HCS) Research Collaboratory, which encourages partnerships between health care delivery systems rather than relying on single research centers (Matthews, 2012; NIH, 2012b). The Collaboratory enhances "the national capacity to implement cost-effective large-scale research studies" (NIH, 2012b). In 2010 the Patient-Centered Outcomes Research Institute was established to provide the best available evidence to help patients and their health care providers make more informed decisions (Burns, 2012; PCORI, 2013). These new entities and collaborations are bridging gaps between research and practice in ways that could expedite the translational process.

Community engagement is becoming an established principle in facilitating and strengthening clinical research (Task Force on the Principles of Community Engagement, 2011; Zerhouni, 2005). Government, patients, families, and advocacy groups are increasingly recognizing the value of community engagement. As a result, patient advocacy groups, health care providers, and community organizations are assuming more active roles in processes related to peer review, research protocol design, recruitment and retention of participants in clinical research, and translation of findings back to the community. Studies of broader community involvement could strengthen evidence of the value of community participation and provide best practices of community engagement across all phases of clinical and translational research.

Emerging Data and Technology

The public- and private-sectors are further increasing access to new sources of health-related data and forging new partnerships to revolutionize the way this information is disseminated and used. For example, the Health Data Initiative, launched in 2010 by HHS and the IOM, "is a public–private collaboration that encourages innovators to utilize health data to develop applications to raise awareness of health and health system performance and spark community action to improve health" (IOM, 2013b).

Advances in computational abilities and connectivity, as well as implementation of EHRs, are facilitating many clinical and translational research projects. Each year, the capacity to share information rises by approximately 30 percent (Hilbert and López, 2011; IOM, 2011). New developments in bioinformatics allow researchers to store, retrieve, organize, protect, and analyze vast amounts of data, resulting in larger and more efficient clinical research and trials (CTSA PIs, 2012). This capacity is enhanced by developing technologies, such as "mobile and social computing with advanced analytics to enable fact-based decision-making" (Cognizant, 2012b, p. 5). These rapidly changing technologies hold great promise for drug development and first-in-human studies (Melese et al., 2009; Waldman and Terzic, 2010).

Data and computational capabilities are "expanding the reach of knowledge, increasing access to clinical information when and where needed, and assisting patients and providers in managing chronic diseases" (IOM, 2013a, p. 15). Health information technology also has the potential to improve the quality and efficiency of the care that patients receive, through improved diagnostic practices and personalized medicine (Friedman et al., 2010). For example, in Arkansas, Blue Health Intelligence is applying predictive analytics to claims databases in order to reduce costs by improving the care of patients with diabetes (Rosenbush, 2012). EHRs, now used by more than half of all physicians in the United States (Jamoom et al., 2012), enable HMOs, PBRNs, and other research networks to serve as venues and partners for patient-oriented research (e.g., comparative-effectiveness research) (Elliott, 2012; Miriovsky et al., 2012). In addition, studies are currently investigating the potential usefulness of EHRs in improving patient participation in their care and overall outcomes (University of Illinois at Urbana-Champaign, 2011).

Streamlined IRB Review Processes and Enhanced Patient Protections

Increased coordination between a growing number of private and public institutions has led to streamlined research oversight while enhancing patient protections. In compliance with federal regulations governing human subject research,[3] a number of multisite studies are choosing to use single IRBs to coordinate joint, multi-institution IRB review of research protocols. For example, the Central Institutional Review Board Initiative performs a single review of some National Cancer Institute–sponsored multicenter protocols, allowing the local IRB to focus solely on ethical issues unique to local conditions (Millum and Menikoff, 2010). The CTSA Consortium's IRBshare system facilitates multisite studies by using shared review documents that are supported by a centralized secure Web portal and an IRBshare Master Agreement (Vanderbilt University, 2013).

New approaches to clinical trial monitoring also strengthen research participant protections. In response to increasingly variable investigator experience, ethical oversight, site infrastructure, health care standards, treatment choices, and the globalization of clinical research (Glickman et al., 2009), many study sponsors are capitalizing on new technologies and strategies to enhance the efficiency and effectiveness of monitoring activities. For example, centralized monitoring allows sponsor organizations to assess data trends and access data remotely to identify deviations or problems more efficiently (Bhatt, 2011; Cognizant, 2012a; FDA,

---

[3]45 C.F.R. 46.

2011). Moreover, risk-based monitoring verifies completion of critical study parameters that protect human research participants while maintaining study integrity (FDA, 2011).

Broader Research Participant Recruitment

Research participant recruitment efforts have increased and diversified in response to persistent barriers to enrollment and retention of research participants. Research participants now include individuals in randomized trials, patients and their records within health care networks, and collaborating institutions and community organizations. As noted by Harris and colleagues (2012), however, the general public has little knowledge about clinical research or how to participate, despite an interest in clinical trials. ResearchMatch, a CTSA-developed tool, was created to overcome recruitment challenges by connecting volunteers and researchers. In its first 19 months, approximately half of the studies that used ResearchMatch were clinical trials. Other types of research using ResearchMatch include behavioral and psychosocial studies, observational studies, and community-based research (Harris et al., 2012). Collaborations between CTSAs and organizations such as PBRNs, are also working to engage a wide range of community members across the entire clinical research process, including clinical research participant recruitment (NCATS, 2012).

Development of a Dynamic Research Workforce

The continued success of clinical and translational research depends on an adaptable, well-trained, and diverse workforce. As the field of translational science continues to evolve, so too must programs continue to update the skills of the existing workforce as well as prepare the next generation of scientists and clinicians. Demographic shifts in the U.S. population require a strong commitment to achieving greater participation of underrepresented groups in clinical and translational research careers at both the investigator and patient care levels. Effective clinical and translational research requires teams of researchers that can traverse the divides between basic and clinical sciences and health care practice. Key members of these teams will be clinician-scientists. The proportion of physicians involved in research has declined steadily in recent decades, however, and innovative solutions and incentives are needed to reverse this trend (Roberts et al., 2012). Investments in interdisciplinary training and mentoring programs continue to be a core function of the CTSA Program, offering opportunities to bolster the research workforce. Continuous innovations are necessary to encourage multidisciplinary, team-based science—a core CTSA principle (Kroenke et al., 2010; Pienta et al., 2011).

A VISION FOR THE CTSA PROGRAM

Despite the accelerating pace of scientific discovery, the current clinical research enterprise does not adequately tackle pressing clinical and methodological questions relevant to health and health care improvement. CTSAs can play a substantial role in facilitating efforts to remediate limitations in the clinical and translational research ecosystem such as the following: challenges associated with first-in-human studies; limited recruitment and retention in clinical trials; the identification and measurement of health outcomes to assess intervention effectiveness; barriers to increasing awareness about research resources and potential research partnerships at the investigator and community levels; lack of incentives for team-based science; policy and regulatory challenges in developing full and substantive collaborations with industry and other partners; and ethical concerns (including related regulatory requirements) associated with the interplay between clinical research and practice.

The CTSA Program has been successful in establishing CTSAs as academic focal points for clinical and translational research. Its 61 awardees can have a broad impact on research practices and informatics and, ultimately, on patient care and individual health outcomes. The CTSAs continue to provide funding and infrastructure to investigators in their local environments, facilitating the conduct of clinical and transla-tional research and the training of the translational science workforce. In addition, the CTSA Program has begun to foster interactions with the community and outside partners, such as the pharmaceutical industry.

Yet, more progress is needed in order to assure a proactive research environment responsive to the demands of a continually evolving health care landscape. As the new home for the CTSA Program, NCATS has described a commitment to building on the program's initial accomplishments with further advances. NCATS has called the next phase of the program CTSA 2.0 (Briggs and Austin, 2012), a term the IOM committee has adopted and uses in this report. The challenge for this next phase of the CTSA Program will be to set the goals and create the incentives for these 61 sites to function as the core of a national network that initiates and sustains collaborations both inside and outside their home institutions, across NIH institutes and centers, and with community, industry, and research network partners.

The IOM committee envisions a transformation of the CTSA Program from its current, loosely organized structure into a more tightly integrated network, with all the sites, committees, and coordinating center working collectively to enhance the transit of therapeutics, diagnostics, and preventive interventions along the developmental pipeline; disseminate innovative translational research methods and best practices; and provide leadership in informatics standards and policy development to promote shared resources. By providing infrastructure and innovations to accelerate clinical and translational research, an increasingly networked CTSA Program will increase its benefit to research and researchers across diseases, health conditions, age ranges, and health care delivery systems.

To reach its potential in an ever-changing environment, the CTSA Program must build on its core strengths and successes and transform CTSAs from academic research homes to active hubs in a fully integrated network of clinical and translational research. On the basis of its findings, the IOM committee identified four key opportunities for action to guide efforts to strengthen the CTSA Program and ensure future success:

- *Adopt and sustain active program leadership*—NCATS should increase its leadership presence in the overall program, consistent with the cooperative agreement model under which the CTSAs are funded. A centralized leadership model that includes participation by NCATS, leaders of individual CTSAs, community partners, and other stakeholders will increase overall program efficiency, enable mechanisms for maximizing accountability, and provide the direction needed to develop and nurture substantive partnerships.
- *Engage in substantive and productive collaborations*—The CTSA Program needs to capitalize on the collaborations developed within and among individual CTSAs and continue to initiate and forge true partnerships with other NIH institutes and centers and with entities external to the program, including

patient groups, communities, health care providers, industry, and regulatory organizations.

- *Develop and widely disseminate innovative research resources*—Fully developing the role of the CTSA Program as a facilitator and accelerator of clinical and translational research will require enhanced efforts to engage and support researchers and other stakeholders as they develop, refine, widely disseminate, and implement novel research and health informatics tools, methodologies, policies, and other resources.

- *Build on initial successes in training and education, community engagement, and child health research*—The CTSA Program needs to continue its strong efforts in each of these areas. A robust and diverse workforce that is well trained in team science is critically important. Ensuring an emphasis on community involvement across the research spectrum will bring a range of much-needed perspectives and innovations along with increased public support for research. Program efforts can also help overcome the paucity of research specific to child health.

REFERENCES

Austin, C. P. 2013. *National Center for Advancing Translational Sciences: Catalyzing translational innovation.* PowerPoint presented at Meeting 3: IOM Committee to Review the CTSA Program at NCATS, Washington, DC, January 24. http://www.iom.edu/~/media/Files/Activity%20Files/Research/CTSAReview/2013-JAN-24/Chris%20Austin.pdf (accessed February 13, 2013).

Bhatt, A. 2011. Quality of clinical trials: A moving target. *Perspectives in Clinical Research* 2(4):115–150.

Briggs, J., and C. P. Austin. 2012. *NCATS and the evolution of the Clinical and Translational Science Award (CTSA) Program.* PowerPoint presented at Meeting 1: IOM Committee to Review the CTSA Program at NCATS, Washington, DC, October 29. http://www.iom.edu/~/media/Files/Activity%20Files/Research/CTSAReview/2012-OCT-29/IOM%20Briggs-Austin%20102912.pdf (accessed February 13, 2013).

Burns, J. 2012. What works best for patients? PCORI hopes to provide answers. *Managed Care*, December: 36–39. http://www.managedcaremag.com/archives/1212/1212.pcori.html (accessed February 13, 2013).

Butler, D. 2008. Translational research: Crossing the valley of death. *Nature* 453(12):840–842.

Calmbach, W. L., J. G. Ryan, L.-M. Baldwin, and L. Knox. 2012. Practice-Based Research Networks (PBRNs): Meeting the challenges of the future. *Journal of the American Board of Family Medicine* 25(5):572–576.

Casagrande, S. S., J. E. Fradkin, S. H. Saydah, K. F. Rust, and C. C. Cowie. 2013. The prevalence of meeting A1C, blood pressure, and LDL goals among people with diabetes, 1988–2010. *Diabetes Care*, February 15. http://care.diabetesjournals.org/content/early/2013/02/07/dc12-2258.full.pdf+html (accessed April 3, 2013).

CFF (Cystic Fibrosis Foundation). 2013. *Cystic Fibrosis Foundation therapeutics.* http://www.cff.org/research/cfft (accessed May 6, 2013).

Chappel, R. J., K. M. Wilson, and E. M. Dax. 2009. Immunoassays for the diagnosis of HIV: Meeting future needs by enhancing the quality of testing. *Future Microbiology* 4(8):963–982.

Cognizant. 2012a. *Cognizant's clinical transformation: More than a solution, it's a new way to work.* http://www.cognizant.com/OurApproach/Cognizants-Clinical-Transformation-More%20-Than-Solution-Its-a-New-Way-to-Work.pdf (accessed April 10, 2013).

———. 2012b. *A vision for U.S. healthcare's radical makeover.* http://www.cognizant.com/InsightsWhitepapers/A-Vision-for-US-Health-Radical-Makeover.pdf (accessed March 28, 2013).

Commonwealth Fund. 2011. *Why not the best? Results from the National Scorecard on U.S. Health System Performance, 2011.* Washington, DC: Commonwealth Fund. http://www.commonwealthfund.org/~/media/Files/Publications/Fund%20Report/2011/Oct/1500_WNTB_Natl_Scorecard_2011_web.pdf (accessed March 26, 2013).

CTSA PIs (Clinical and Translational Science Awards Principal Investigators). 2012. Preparedness of the CTSA's structural and scientific assets to support the mission of the National Center for Advancing Translational Sciences (NCATS). *Clinical and Translational Science* 5(2):121–129.

Elliott, V. S. 2012. Practices can use EMRs to join more clinical trials. *AMA News.* http://www.ama-assn.org/amednews/2012/03/12/bica0312.htm (accessed February 13, 2013).

EMBL-EBI (European Molecular Biology Laboratory-European Bioinformatics Institute). 2013. *1000 Genomes Project.* http://www.1000genomes.org/data (accessed May 7, 2013).

Faden, R. R., N. E. Kass, S. N. Goodman, P. Pronovost, S. Tunis, and T. L. Beauchamp. 2013. An ethics framework for a learning health care system: A departure from traditional research ethics and clinical ethics. *Hastings Center Special Report* 43(1):s16–s27.

FDA (Food and Drug Administration). 2011. *Guidance for industry: Oversight of clinical investigations—a risk-based approach to monitoring: Draft guidance.* Rockville, MD: FDA. http://www.fda.gov/downloads/Drugs/.../Guidances/UCM269919.pdf (accessed April 10, 2013).

————. 2012. *FDA approves first over-the-counter home-use rapid HIV test.* http://www.fda.gov/NewsEvents/Newsroom/PressAnnouncements/ucm310 542.htm (accessed April 3, 2013).

Friedman, C. P., A. K. Wong, and D. Blumenthal. 2010. Achieving a nationwide learning health system. *Science Translational Medicine* 2(57):1–3.

Fries, J., M. Rose, and E. Krishnan. 2011. The PROMIS of better outcome assessment: Responsiveness, floor and ceiling effects, and Internet administration. *Journal of Rheumatology* 38(8):1759–1764.

Fulda, K. G., K. A. Hahn, R. A. Young, J. D. Marshall, B. J. Moore, A. M. Espinoza, N. M. Beltran, P. McFadden, A. D. Crim, and R. Cardarelli. 2011. Recruiting Practice-based Research Network (PBRN) physicians to be research participants: Lessons learned from the North Texas (NorTex) needs assessment study. *Journal of the American Board of Family Medicine* 24(5):610–615.

Glickman, S. W., J. G. McHutchison, E. D. Peterson, C. B. Cairns, R. A. Harrington, R. M. Califf, and K. A. Schulman. 2009. Ethical and scientific implications of the globalization of clinical research. *New England Journal of Medicine* 360(8):816–823.

Harris, P. A., K. W. Scott, L. Lebo, N. Hassan, C. Lightner, and J. Pulley. 2012. ResearchMatch: A national registry to recruit volunteers for clinical research. *Academic Medicine* 87(1):66–73.

Hilbert, M., and P. López. 2011. The world's technological capacity to store, communicate, and compute information. *Science* 332(6025):60–65.

IOM (Institute of Medicine). 1998. *Statement on quality of care.* Washington, DC: National Academy Press.

————. 2001. *Crossing the quality chasm: A new health system for the 21st century.* Washington, DC: National Academy Press.

————. 2010. *Clinical data as the basic staple of health learning: Creating and protecting a public good: Workshop summary.* Washington, DC: The National Academies Press.

————. 2011. Visioning perspectives on the digital health utility. Chapter 2. In *Digital infrastructure for the learning health system: The foundation for continuous improvement in health and health care: Workshop series summary.* Washington, DC: The National Academies Press.

————. 2013a. *Best care at lower cost: The path to continuously learning health care in America.* Washington, DC: The National Academies Press.

————. 2013b. *The health data initiative.* http://www.iom.edu/Activities/ PublicHealth/HealthData.aspx (accessed March 28, 2013).

————. 2013c. *Sharing clinical research data: Workshop summary.* Washington, DC: The National Academies Press.

Jamoom, E., P. Beatty, A. Bercovitz, D. Woodwell, K. Palso, and E. Rechtsteiner. 2012. *Physician adoption of electronic health record systems: United States, 2011.* Hyattsville, MD: National Center for Health Statistics. http://www.cdc.gov/nchs/data/databriefs/db98.htm (accessed April 3, 2013).

Kemp, K. B. 2012. *Research insights: Using evidence to build a learning health care system.* Washington, DC: AcademyHealth. http://www.academy health.org/files/publications/AHUsingEvidence2012.pdf (accessed April 10, 2013).

Kroenke, K., W. Kapoor, M. Helfand, D. O. Meltzer, M. A. McDonald, H. Selker, and CTSA Consortium Strategic Goal Committee on Comparative Effectiveness Research: Workgroup on Workforce Development. 2010. Training and career development for comparative effectiveness research workforce development. *Clinical and Translational Science* 3(5):258–262.

Larson, E. B., C. Tachibana, and E. H. Wagner. 2013. Sparking and sustaining the essential fuctions of research: What supports translation of research into health care? Answers from the Group Health experience. In *Enhancing the professional culture of academic health science centers: The organizational environment and its impact on research*, edited by T. S. Inui and R. M. Frankel. London, UK: Radcliffe.

Lieu, T. A., V. L. Hinrichsen, A. Moreira, and R. Platt. 2011. Collaborations in population-based health research. *Clinical Medicine and Research* 9(3/4):137–140.

Main, D. S., M. C. Felzien, D. J. Magid, B. N. Calonge, R. A. O'Brien, A. Kempe, and K. Nearing. 2012. A community translational research pilot grants program to facilitate community-academic partnerships: Lessons from Colorado's Clinical Translational Science Awards. *Progress in Community Health Partnerships: Research, Education, and Action* 6(3):381–387.

Marantz, P. R., A. H. Strelnick, B. Currie, R. Bhalla, A. E. Blank, P. Meissner, P. A. Selwyn, E. A. Walker, D. T. Hsu, and H. Shamoon. 2011. Developing a multidisciplinary model of comparative effectiveness research within a Clinical and Translational Science Award. *Academic Medicine* 86(6):712–717.

Matthews, S. 2012. New NIH effort seeks to find ways to make trials run smoother. *Nature Medicine* 18(11):1598.

Melese, T., S. M. Lin, J. L. Chang, and N. H. Cohen. 2009. Open innovation networks between academia and industry: An imperative for breakthrough therapies. *Nature Medicine* 15(5):502–507.

Millum, J., and J. Menikoff. 2010. Streamlining ethical review. *Annals of Internal Medicine* 153(10):655–657.

Miriovsky, B. J., L. N. Shulman, and A. P. Abernethy. 2012. Importance of health information technology, electronic health records, and continuously aggregating data to comparative effectiveness research and learning health care. *Journal of Clinical Oncology* 30(34):4243–4248.

NCATS (National Center for Advancing Translational Sciences). 2012. *Request for information: Enhancing the Clinical and Translational Science Awards Program.* http://www.ncats.nih.gov/files/report-ctsa-rfi.pdf (accessed April 8, 2013).

NIH (National Institutes of Health). 2012a. *1000 Genomes Project available on Amazon Cloud.* http://www.nih.gov/news/health/mar2012/nhgri-29.htm (accessed April 3, 2013).

———. 2012b. NIH funds will strengthen national capacity for cost-effective, large-scale clinical studies. *NIH News.* hhtp://www.nih.gov/news/health/sep2012/nccam-25.htm (accessed February 13, 2013).

NIH PROMIS (Patient Reported Outcomes Measurement Information Systems). 2013. *PROMIS: Patient Reported Outcomes Measurement Information Systems.* http://www.nihpromis.org (accessed February 13, 2013).

PCORI (Patient-Centered Outcomes Research Institute). 2013. *Patient-Centered Outcomes Research Institute (PCORI): About us.* http://www.pcori.org/about-us (accessed February 13, 2013).

Pfizer. 2013. *Centers for Therapeutic Innovation.* http://www.pfizer.com/research/rd_works/centers_for_therapeutic_innovation.jsp (accessed May 6, 2013).

Pienta, K. J., J. Scheske, and A. L. Spork. 2011. The Clinical and Translational Science Awards (CTSAs) are transforming the way academic medical institutions approach translational research: The University of Michigan experience. *Clinical and Translational Science* 4(4):233–235.

Porter, M. E. 2010. What is value in health care? *New England Journal of Medicine* 363(26):2477–2481.

Porter, M. E., and E. O. Teisberg. 2006. *Redefining health care: Creating value-based competition on results.* Cambridge, MA: Harvard Business School Press.

Pritts, J. L. 2008. *The importance and value of protecting the privacy of health information: The roles of the HIPAA Privacy Rule and the Common Rule in health research.* Commissioned by the Committee on Health Research and the Privacy of Health Information, Washington, DC: Institute of Medicine. http://www.iom.edu/~/media/Files/Activity%20Files/Research/HIPAA andResearch/PrittsPrivacyFinalDraftweb.ashx (accessed May 7, 2013).

Reed, J. C., E. L. White, J. Aube, C. Lindsley, M. Li, L. Sklar, and S. Schreiber. 2012. The NIH's role in accelerating translational sciences. *Nature Biotechnology* 30(1):16–19.

Roberts, S. F., M. A. Fischhoff, S. A. Sakowski, and E. L. Feldman. 2012. Perspective: Transforming science into medicine: How clinician-scientists can build bridges across research's "valley of death." *Academic Medicine* 87(3):266–270.

Rosenbush, S. 2012. Blue Cross expects costs savings from big data dive. *CIO Journal,* March 30, 2012. http://mobile.blogs.wsj.com/cio/2012/03/30/blue-cross-expects-cost-savings-from-big-data-dive (accessed May 7, 2013).

Shuster, J. J. 2012. U.S. government mandates for clinical and translational research. *Clinical and Translational Science* 5(1):83–84.

Task Force on the Principles of Community Engagement (Clinical and Translational Science Awards Consortium Community Engagement Key Function Committee Task Force on the Principles of Community

Engagement). 2011. *Principles of community engagement: Second edition.* NIH Publication No. 11-7782. http://www.atsdr.cdc.gov/community engagement/pdf/PCE_Report_508_FINAL.pdf (accessed April 2, 2013).

University of Illinois at Urbana-Champaign. 2011. *Medtable: An electronic medical record strategy to promote patient medication understanding and use, NCT01296633.* http://www.clinicaltrials.gov/ct2/show/NCT01296633? term=medtable&rank=1 (accessed February 13, 2013).

Vanderbilt University. 2013. *IRBshare.* https://www.irbshare.org (accessed February 13, 2013).

Waldman, S. A., and A. Terzic. 2010. Molecular therapy drives patient-centric healthcare paradigms. *Clinical and Translational Science* 3(4):170–171.

Zerhouni, E. A. 2005. Translational and clinical science—time for a new vision. *New England Journal of Medicine* 353(15):1621–1623.

3

Leadership

As envisioned by the Institute of Medicine (IOM) committee, the Clinical and Translational Science Awards (CTSA) Program has the potential to overcome many bottlenecks and pioneer new solutions that can be used to accelerate clinical and translational research. Accomplishing the tasks ahead, however, will require a revitalized approach to program leadership—one that builds on the academic homes that have been established and moves toward an integrated network of CTSAs that increasingly applies collaborative and systems-based approaches. Leadership opportunities and challenges facing the CTSA Program are outlined in this chapter with discussion and recommendations related to leadership strategies, organizational structure, collaborations and partnerships, leadership for individual CTSAs, evaluation, and communications. Leading the CTSA Program into its next phase, CTSA 2.0, will involve building on the strengths of individual CTSAs; leveraging the dedication of individuals working in clinical and translational science; and expanding successful collaborative endeavors, both within and outside of the National Institutes of Health (NIH).

LEADERSHIP STRATEGIES

Balancing the tensions and benefits of two seemingly contradictory approaches to leadership is one of the challenges inherent in an endeavor with the scope and structure of the CTSA Program. A variety of possible advantages and disadvantages exist for differing leadership approaches. For example, the grass-roots approach to leadership offers the potential for creativity and innovation. It harnesses the dedication and energy of multiple researchers and stakeholders, all with an interest in moving clinical and translational research forward, but all of whom also have ties and obligations to their home institutions. The top-down leadership approach offers the potential for a systems-level perspective, greater focus and direction, and a commitment to progress for the overall research enterprise. However, this approach usually means fewer people will have direct decision-making responsibilities, and it requires careful oversight and coordination to ensure that multiple people and projects are on track and working to meet the same goals. Finding the correct balance between these two approaches will be an important element for future CTSA success.

As CTSA 2.0 moves forward, the IOM committee sees the need for a more centralized approach to leadership, one in which National Center for Advancing Translational Sciences (NCATS) plays a more active role. To date, the program has, for the most part, relied on the energy and efforts of individual CTSAs and their principal investigators (PIs). This has created a largely ad hoc structure and process for identifying next steps and overall management. Direction from the NIH (first through the National Center for Research Resources [NCRR] and more recently through NCATS) has been articulated primarily through the funding announcements. With each cycle of applications for new CTSAs or renewals, these announcements have emphasized specific key functions or priorities for the investigators to include in their applications.

The mechanism by which the CTSA Program is funded gives NCATS the opportunity to lead awardees toward fulfilling the NIH's vision for the program both in the performance of individual institutions and in the program's overall achievements. The NIH has three funding mechanisms for making research awards—grants, contracts, and cooperative agreements. The individual CTSAs and the coordinating center are funded through cooperative agreements. The salient feature of cooperative agreements is that NIH staff members provide assistance to awardees "above and beyond the levels usually required for program stewardship of grants. This level of stewardship is known as substantial involvement" (OIG, 2011, p. i). Substantial involvement can be achieved through various means, including technical assistance, advice, and coordination, and the most recent request for applications (RFA) for the CTSA Program noted that "substantial involvement means that, after award, NIH staff will assist, guide, coordinate, or participate in project activities" (NIH, 2012c).

Cooperative agreements provide the structure and mechanisms with which NCATS can exert a stronger leadership role while also promoting collaboration and innovation by individual CTSAs and researchers and guiding the program forward. As described throughout this chapter, the IOM committee urges NCATS to take a more active role in the direction and oversight of the CTSA Program. A number of lessons can be learned from a report on the program's early experience that was prepared by the Department of Health and Human Services' (HHS's) Office of the Inspector General (OIG) (discussed below), as well from insights gained from the management of other collectives of academic institutions working toward specific goals, such as the Human Genome Project (HGP). Although there are several differences between the HGP and the CTSA Program, they share many common elements, such as the following:

- an emphasis on innovation, supported by the development of new technologies and databases;
- the expectation of useful, actionable results and a need for ongoing evaluation;
- an emphasis on efficiency and timely outcomes;
- the development of a parallel research effort in bioethics and, in the CTSA case, community involvement; and
- a commitment to collaborative, team-based science and to widely sharing tools and results.

An analysis of the management of HGP identified five key factors in the project's success. HGP had (1) a clear goal; (2) a flexible organizational structure (the "bottom-up" approach); (3) political support; (4) competition; and (5) strong leadership (the "top-down" approach) (Lambright, 2002). The Lambright analysis of the program says that, of these factors, "the fifth was the most important because it pulled the other factors together and made the most of them when it counted" (2002, p. 5). Leadership manifested in different ways over the life of the project and ultimately provided a balance between the top-down and bottom-up leadership approaches that not only promoted flexibility and innovation but also provided the direction and oversight needed to achieve outcomes.

Although the purpose and tasks of the two programs were widely different, a number of management and leadership lessons can be learned from the HGP that could be useful in the administration of the CTSA Program. For example, as with the HGP, a compelling vision, clearly articulated goals, and a mission-oriented approach could be used to organize and align the work of the individual CTSAs. In addition, the combination of flexibility and active leadership that was used in the HGP to promote innovation and excellence in a pool of talented, multidisciplinary researchers collaborating across multiple research centers is also applicable to the CTSA Program.

Although collaboration was a key element of the HGP, the types of collaboration and partnerships necessary to define and achieve success for the CTSA Program are very different (e.g., community partnerships, collaboration with industry) and will require new leadership strategies.

In 2011, the HHS OIG conducted a review of the administration of the CTSA Program in which OIG reviewers assessed files for the 38 cooperative agreements awarded from 2006 through 2008 (when the program was administered by the NCRR). This assessment found numerous lapses in program oversight. In addition to the administrative critiques described in the report, the OIG found no evidence that NIH program staff provided the "substantial involvement" required by federal regulations and NIH policy with respect to cooperative agreements. In fact, OIG reviewers found no documentation of technical assistance by project scientists for any of the cooperative agreements. Further, they found no evidence that project scientists assisted awardees in performing project activities; stopped activities that were not meeting performance requirements; reviewed or approved the various stages of projects; approved the selection of key personnel, subawardees, or external contractors; conducted technical monitoring; or served on committees (OIG, 2011). The NCRR agreed that relevant information was not in the files in a meaningful way and presented its view that the NCRR worked with awardees "jointly in a partner role but did not assume direction, prime responsibility, or a dominant role" (OIG, 2011, p. 27). Although more project monitoring and aid may have taken place than the files reflect, there is no way to know. The OIG made several recommendations to remedy these shortcomings, including the following:

- "NIH must ensure that staff document awardee accomplishments toward meeting project goals; reasons for not meeting project goals, if applicable; and plans for activities during the coming year."
- "NIH should ensure that staff document correspondence with awardees as they act to obtain delinquent progress reports and financial status reports."
- "At a minimum, staff must clearly list the Project Scientists involved and include the annual summary of involvement within the award files" (OIG, 2011, pp. ii–iii).

In considering the next steps for the CTSA Program and the recommendations that are made in this report, the IOM committee believes that NCATS should learn from previous experiences and lessons and take a more active role in the direction and oversight of the CTSA Program. The goal would be to ensure the highest achievable performance of individual CTSAs and to provide stronger guidance toward the development of a national network of institutions engaged in accelerating clinical and translational science. As the program's newly designated home, NCATS has the opportunity, mission, and purpose to provide leadership for CTSA 2.0 and subsequent program phases.

In addition to setting program direction through a revised mission and strategic goals for the CTSA Program (described in the following section), more active NCATS leadership will require that it take on significant responsibilities in promoting collaborations, conducting evaluations of progress, and ensuring that the program leverages the innovations provided by each of the individual CTSAs and their researchers, leaders, staff, and partners. Striking the right balance between top-down and grass-roots leadership will not be easy, and a number of challenges and possible unintended consequences need to be carefully considered as changes are made to the governance and leadership of the program. For example, imposing a top-down generated research agenda or priorities that do not meet the needs of local researchers, health care providers, and communities would conflict with the original intent and spirit of the program. In addition, an overly directive approach to leadership could dampen creativity, ingenuity, and collaboration among the on-the-ground researchers. More active, but appropriately balanced, leadership from NCATS, combined with the creative talents and leadership from the PIs, will be critical in moving the CTSA Program to a more systems- and network-based approach to clinical and translational research and ensuring that the program remains focused on the outcomes most relevant to its overarching mission.

Given the size of the CTSA Program, appropriate feedback loops and checks and balances should be incorporated into the program's governance, particularly through the vice-chair and other PIs on the new steering committee that is recommended below. These bidirectional communication and governance strategies will help achieve balanced and informed leadership and will ensure that the active engagement of the on-the-ground perspectives and expertise is maintained and promoted.

Defining the Mission and Goals of the CTSA Program

When NCATS was created in December 2011, components of various NIH programs were moved into the new center. These components include the CTSA Program, the Office of Rare Diseases Research, a variety of programs and activities that are housed in the NCATS Office of the Director for re-engineering translational research,[1] and the newly created Cures Acceleration Network (IOM, 2012; NCATS, 2013c). All of these diverse activities must work together in order to fulfill the NCATS mission. Maximizing the benefits of bringing these various elements together within NCATS requires rethinking the missions and goals of the individual pieces. The need for greater alignment within and across HHS agencies and activities was a major theme of a 2009 IOM report, *HHS in the 21st Century: Charting a New Course for a Healthier America*, which concluded that better alignment and focus on performance were essential to meeting departmental and agency goals (IOM, 2009).

Mission

As the CTSA Program matures, it is important to revisit the missions of NCATS and the CTSA Program to ensure alignment and that the CTSA Program supports the mission of NCATS. This IOM committee was specifically asked for its assessment of the appropriateness of the CTSA Program's mission and goals. Box 3-1 contains the current mission statements of NIH, NCATS, and the CTSA Program. In considering the appropriateness of the CTSA mission, the committee heard both support for preserving coverage of the full spectrum of clinical and translational research from T0–T4 and concern about the feasibility of doing so, given the limited available resources (IOM, 2013a). Tension about the scope of mission and uncertainty about the adequacy of resources is also reflected in the input that NIH received, in response to a request for information (RFI), regarding ways to improve the program (Mulligan, 2012; NCATS, 2012c).

The IOM committee noted that the current mission of NCATS could be interpreted as being more narrowly focused on the development of diagnostics and therapeutics than on the more global mission of the

---

[1] For example, the tissue chip for drug screening initiative, activities related to rescuing and repurposing drugs, and activities related to identifying and validating drug targets.

BOX 3-1
Aligning the Missions

Current Mission Statements

NIH Mission: to seek fundamental knowledge about the nature and behavior of living systems and the application of that knowledge to enhance health, lengthen life, and reduce the burdens of illness and disability.

NCATS Mission: to catalyze the generation of innovative methods and technologies that will enhance the development, testing, and implementation of diagnostics and therapeutics across a wide range of human diseases and conditions.

CTSA Current Program Mission: seeks to strengthen the full spectrum of translational research. Institutional CTSA awards are the centerpiece of the program, providing academic homes for translational sciences and supporting research resources needed by local and national research communities to improve the quality and efficiency of all phases of translational research. Institutional CTSAs also support the training of clinical and translational scientists and the development of all disciplines needed for a robust workforce for translational research.

Proposed CTSA Program Mission Statement

A Suggested Streamlined Mission: to improve the quality and efficiency of the full spectrum of clinical and translational research and to speed the development and use of new diagnostics, therapeutics, and preventive interventions.

SOURCES: NCATS, 2013a,b; NIH, 2011.

CTSA Program, which focuses on the full spectrum of clinical and translational research including preventive interventions and translation into front-line clinical and community practice. The committee concurs with NCATS's recent decision to allow increased flexibility for individual CTSAs in meeting program requirements, while ensuring that the CTSA Program as a whole continues to support the full spectrum of clinical and translational research.

The current CTSA Program mission statement conflates mission and goals. As indicated below, strategic goals should be separated from the mission, and both need to be clear and consistent. The most recent RFA refers to a slightly different mission than that shown in Box 3-1, stating that the program works toward "increased quality, efficiency, and decreased cost of all translational research within academic institutions and nationally" (NIH, 2012c).

A revamping of the mission should strive for simplicity and should reflect the program's overarching purpose. In working to update the mission of the CTSA Program, the committee suggests that NCATS also consider whether revisions to its own mission statement would help achieve better alignment between the two missions, highlighting support for the full spectrum of clinical and translational research. The committee's suggested streamlined mission for the CTSA Program also is provided in Box 3-1.

Goals

Although the difference between mission and goals may seem largely semantic, the lack of separately articulated, achievable goals—versus a broad mission—weakens the ability to measure overall progress and establish accountability. As the CTSA Program has grown and evolved, variations on the goals have been cited, which indicates the goals of the program have not been communicated consistently and may not be well understood. For example, a CTSA fact sheet notes that "its goals are to accelerate the translation of laboratory discoveries into treatments for patients, to engage communities in clinical research efforts, and to train a new generation of clinical and translational researchers" (NCATS, 2012a), and the recent RFA said that "the goal of the CTSA Program remains focused on integrated academic homes for the clinical and translational sciences that increase the quality, safety, efficiency and speed of clinical and translational research, particularly for NIH supported research" (NIH, 2012c). Most recently, the program's website describes goals for the "next phase" of the CTSA Program:

- "Building a better bridge between pre-clinical and clinical science;
- Providing a foundation of shared resources that could reduce costs, delays and difficulties experienced in clinical research, including trials;
- Developing partnerships for research to be better integrated across sites and into ongoing patient care; and
- Strengthening strategies for engaging patient communities into the research process" (NCATS, 2013b).

The issue of CTSA goals is further complicated by the CTSA Consortium's separate set of five strategic goals:

1. National clinical and translational research capability;
2. Training and career development of clinical and translational scientists;
3. Consortiumwide collaborations;
4. The health of our communities and the nation; and
5. T1 translational research (CTSA Central, 2013a).

As noted in Chapter 1, these consortium-generated goals were developed through a strategic planning process conducted by the PIs in 2008, with the fifth goal added in 2009 (Disis, 2012; Reis et al., 2010). The IOM committee believes that these goals are overly broad and cannot be easily measured. In addition, because innumerable confounding factors in the clinical and translational ecosystem influence progress in these areas (see Chapter 2), the direct impact of the CTSA Program cannot be assessed. As the various lists of goals have grown apart, it is not clear which set, if any, accurately reflects the current and most pressing challenges facing the clinical and translational research ecosystem or the goals that NCATS has for CTSA 2.0.

Clearly defined, measurable goals directly tied to the mission and work of the CTSA Program will help better align the 61 awardees to achieve the vision for a more integrated network and will provide a basis for evaluation, reporting, and accountability. Clearer communication regarding the goals, as distinct from the mission, also would facilitate program management and increase understanding of the program among its stakeholders.

Reshaping and Reconciling Mission and Goals for the Future

NCATS needs to take a leadership role in shaping the CTSA Program's future by engaging in a strategic planning process in collaboration with the CTSAs to revise the program's mission and establish measurable goals. As noted, the work of the CTSA Program has numerous important audiences and touches people in many domains—researchers, educators, clinicians, health care providers, payers, policy makers, staff in other government departments and agencies (e.g., Department of Veterans Affairs, Agency for Healthcare Research and Quality [AHRQ], Centers for Medicare & Medicaid Services, Patient-

Centered Outcomes Research Institute, and the other NIH institutes and centers), private industry, nonprofit funding agencies, and, ultimately most important, communities, patients, and families. All these groups have a vital interest in achieving a more efficient and rapid clinical and translational research enterprise (see, for example, IOM, 2011), and they should be asked for input during the strategic planning process.

In the transition of the CTSA Program from NCRR to NCATS, the NIH sought internal and external advice through an 11-member NIH working group. This group was asked to "enumerate the roles and capabilities of the CTSAs that could support and enhance the mission of NCATS; identify CTSA needs and priorities; and propose processes for ensuring a smooth transition from the NCRR to NCATS" (Katz et al., 2011). The working group consulted widely with individuals involved in the program in developing its recommendations for a smooth integration. In addition, NIH issued an RFI for input from public stakeholders, NIH personnel, and CTSA PIs that generated 139 responses, mostly from CTSA institutions (Mulligan, 2012; NCATS, 2012c). Conducting such broad-based outreach (as well as using the input already collected as a departure point) might be a useful strategy in assuring that relevant viewpoints about the program's mission and goals are considered.

A particular benefit of the collaborative approach to developing plans for integrating the CTSA program into NCATS was the positive response from the individual CTSAs, which demonstrated their "deep commitment to the NCATS mission," willingness to move forward rapidly, and recognition of new opportunities that NCATS would create, including greater visibility and closer, more transparent working relationships with NIH institutes and centers (CTSA PIs, 2012).

Whatever process is adopted should result in a compelling mission statement and a single set of strategic goals that

- are clearly defined and measurable;
- reflect the full range of clinical and translational research;
- are targeted at overcoming specific, current research challenges and barriers;
- encourage clear decision points (go/no-go decisions) that promote a flexible and dynamically responsive program;
- build on program successes and reinforce areas of progress (e.g., training and education, community engagement, child health);

- are fully supported and consistently communicated by all those involved; and
- can serve as the basis for developing a set of common metrics for evaluating the individual CTSAs and the program as a whole.

All components of the CTSA Program—NCATS, CTSA consortium committees, the CTSA Coordinating Center, individual CTSAs, and the researchers whose work is supported through the program—should be focused on achieving these unified goals. This is essential in order to establish accountability and assess progress, as outlined in *HHS in the 21st Century* (IOM, 2009). As the CTSA Program moves forward, these goals should be reviewed and updated periodically as progress is made, as the research ecosystem continues to evolve, and as population health needs change.

STRUCTURE OF THE CTSA PROGRAM

The CTSA Program has grown rapidly, from 12 sites in 2006 to 61 in 2012. From the program's outset, the NIH and the individual CTSAs have recognized the value of collaboration and the need for a cross-institutional structure to advance the program's efforts; this recognition was the beginning of the vision for a CTSA network. In the early stages of the program, the NIH charged CTSAs with developing a national consortium to promote and implement best practices, policies, and procedures (NIH, 2005). The first funding announcement stated that a National CTSA Consortium Steering Committee should be organized for PIs. In addition, as discussed in Chapter 1, it directed that subcommittees be formed to foster advances in the NIH-identified common themes (e.g., education, informatics, regulation) and that these committees meet annually and have representation from each CTSA (NIH, 2005).

In subsequent years, the CTSA Consortium developed largely as an unfunded grass-roots effort through the commitment and energy of PIs and researchers. It now has three leadership committees (Executive Committee, Steering Committee, and Child Health Oversight Committee); committees charged with making progress on each of the 5 CTSA Consortium strategic goals; 14 key function committees, 10 thematic special interest groups, and numerous working groups and task forces under each of those committees. In total, these committees involve more than 2,000 people (CTSA Central, 2013d; Reis et al., 2010) (see Chapter 1).

A 2011 addition is the CTSA Consortium Coordinating Center, which was awarded to Vanderbilt University through a competitive process (Vanderbilt University, 2011). A variety of collaborative informatics tools have been developed and are being disseminated through the Consortium Coordinating Center. One of the most widely adopted is RED-Cap (Research Electronic Data Capture), a Web-based tool for creating online surveys and databases used in clinical research. Currently, 602 institutional partners in 54 countries actively participate in REDCap (Vanderbilt University, 2013b). Other examples of research tools that are available through the CTSA Program are provided in Table 3-1. The full range of collaborative tools developed through the CTSA Program should be assessed, and those deemed successful can be deployed further in NIH-funded projects, with data being shared as openly and freely as possible.

TABLE 3-1 Examples of Collaborative Tools

ROCKET (Research Organization, Collaboration, and Knowledge Exchange Toolkit)	A Web-based tool that provides a common platform for CTSA institutions to share documents and build web pages. ROCKET is designed to be easy for users to edit and maintain their private workspaces but allows specific pages to be made public in order to share information with a larger audience (CTSA Central, 2013g).
IRBshare	This shared IRB review model for multisite studies provides an established set of review documents and review processes as well as an IRBshare Master Agreement. Twenty-three sites currently use the model, and it is open to new NIH-funded studies (Vanderbilt University, 2013a).
ResearchMatch	An online registry aimed at bringing researchers and volunteers together for health-related research. Volunteers willing to participate in studies complete a questionnaire with their contact information and health history. Registered researchers search the database for individuals who qualify for a particular study. Individuals decide whether to allow ResearchMatch to release their contact information to the researcher. Currently, the service is limited to institutions affiliated with the CTSA Program, and in order to gain access to recruit volunteers, researchers must have IRB approval of their pro-

	posal. More than 35,000 research volunteers are currently registered, and more than 1,600 researchers conducting more than 350 studies at 78 institutions are using this resource (Vanderbilt University, 2012)
eagle-i Network	An openly available online network that anyone can use to search for more than 50,000 biomedical resources at 25 member institutions. Resources available vary from biological specimens and reagents to software and physical laboratory space (Harvard College, 2012).
VIVO	An open-source Web application that allows researchers at seven participating institutions to describe their interests, activities, and accomplishments in order to create groups or networks of people with similar research goals within and across institutions (VIVO, 2013).
CTSA-IP	A website that compiles and publicly shares information on technology, intellectual property, and licensing opportunities available through more than 24 CTSA institutions. The goal is to promote research activity and collaboration opportunities among CTSAs (University of Rochester, 2012).

Opportunities and Next Steps

Moving toward systems- and network-based approaches to resolving the challenges in clinical and translational research will require more hands-on leadership from NCATS than in the past; more focused, streamlined, and efficient centralized leadership of the program; and changes in its structure.

The IOM committee believes that CTSA Program governance should be markedly simplified from the current structure, which involves an executive committee and a steering committee, more than 200 committee members total, and separate monthly conference calls. The IOM committee envisions that the primary governance of the program would reside within a new NCATS-CTSA Steering Committee that would be responsible for

- program oversight and direction;
- trans-CTSA activities;
- collaborative efforts with external partners;
- promotion of collaborative opportunities within and outside the NIH;
- identification, dissemination, and implementation of best practices; and
- implementation of a proposed new innovations fund to promote collaboration with other NIH institutes and centers and external partners.

The steering committee should represent a cooperative program leadership effort between NCATS and the CTSAs that provides strategic direction and guides progress to ensure that individual CTSAs and the program as a whole are fulfilling their revised mission and strategic goals. The committee should be chaired by an NCATS lead staff member, with a CTSA PI as vice-chair, and should have a rotating membership representing diverse CTSA and stakeholder interests to ensure responsive and effective governance. The number of steering committee members should be small enough to enable the committee to be nimble and efficient. This steering committee should oversee the Coordinating Center and a streamlined structure of consortium committees (see Figure 3-1). Development of the specific details of committee membership, responsibilities, and operations should be a joint effort between NCATS and the CTSA PIs and should be part of the strategic planning process. This new governance model centralizes accountability for the program and provides a more active leadership role for NCATS, while enabling focused, stakeholder-based leadership that should fully leverage the experience, creativity, and commitment of the CTSA PIs and other stakeholders. As discussed previously, possible disadvantages to a more active leadership role for NCATS should be considered as the governance and structure of the program evolve.

Streamlining the current consortium committee structure is an urgent need. However, the structure and governance should evolve over the next year or two as a component of the recommended strategic planning process. Only those consortium committees that are most relevant to the program's revised goals and priorities should be retained. The current unwieldy committee setup was perhaps a natural result of the rapid

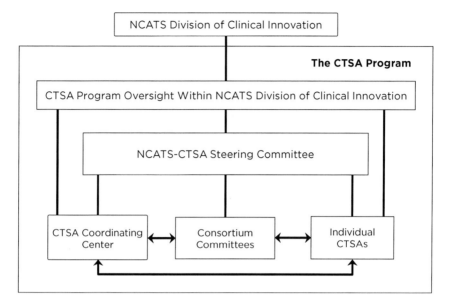

FIGURE 3-1 A revised structure for the CTSA Program in the Division of Clinical Innovation at NCATS. The components of a reorganized CTSA Program would include the staff and CTSA Program oversight activities at NCATS; individual CTSAs; a set of streamlined consortium committees; the CTSA Coordinating Center; and the new NCATS-CTSA Steering Committee, which would provide oversight and direction to the Coordinating Center, the consortium committees, and, to a lesser extent, the individual CTSAs. Leadership, collaboration, and communication among all these entities will be essential for the efficiency and effectiveness of the program overall.

increase in the number of CTSAs, with each wanting to ensure it had a voice in the program's leadership. However, according to testimony received by the IOM committee and from interviews conducted as part of the Westat site visit evaluation, the current number and size of committees—some having more than 150 members—makes too many burdensome demands on researchers' time (Westat, 2011).

While the IOM committee recognizes the dedication and commitment many people have given to the program's work, now is the time to build on what has been accomplished and rechannel that commitment through a leaner structure. The result should be greater management efficiency as well as increased productivity. Larger numbers of stakeholders and CTSA leaders can be convened periodically to communicate progress, solicit input, and plan next steps. With this streamlined structure, care should be taken to ensure that ample opportunities exist for communication; collaboration; and sharing best practices, available resources, and expertise within and across the CTSAs.

Opportunities abound for the CTSA Program to reengineer its structure and governance. A new NCATS-CTSA Steering Committee, along with the Coordinating Center and a simpler consortium committee structure, will position the program to better coordinate the advancement of clinical and translational research.

COLLABORATIONS AND PARTNERSHIPS

The CTSA Program is a facilitator of clinical and translational research. Its inherent function is to initiate and foster collaborations—including developing innovative tools, policies, and processes; removing barriers to research; training teams of investigators; engaging communities in the research process; and other efforts—that bring together researchers, research networks, NIH institutes and centers, community stakeholders, health care providers, industry partners, government research agencies, and others to advance clinical and translational science. NCATS, the CTSA Coordinating Center, and the individual CTSA sites need to ensure that the full range of potential collaborators understands the value that the CTSA Program brings to clinical and translational research and that the Program is responsive to their needs. Incentives for building these partnerships are also needed. The IOM committee urges the establishment of an innovations fund to promote further collaboration and emphasizes that the success of CTSA 2.0 will depend on the extent and strength of the partnerships and collaborations formed.

Collaborations with NIH Institutes and Centers

Some of the most natural partnerships are occurring and need to occur more frequently between the CTSA Program and NIH institutes and centers. A number of NIH institutes and centers have their own research centers, networks, and clinical trials (e.g., Comprehensive Cancer Centers, NeuroNext, Type 1 Diabetes TrialNet) already benefiting from the CTSA Program's collaborative databases and tools. Nonetheless, individuals who provided testimony to the IOM committee reported that intra-NIH collaborations with the CTSA Program need to be strengthened.

Evidence of the potential for collaboration is shown in Figure 3-2, which reports the number of NIH grants using some form of CTSA support or resources, although the extent and depth of that interaction is not indicated. CTSA support or resources frequently come in the form of providing institute grantees with facilities, core resources, equipment, staff expertise, or administrative services. They may also take the form of providing specific tools, such as those described earlier. Box 3-2 illustrates some of the general CTSA resources that NIH institutes are finding helpful.

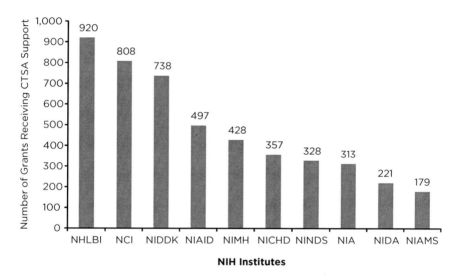

FIGURE 3-2 Top 10 NIH institutes and centers using CTSA resources.
NOTE: NCI = National Cancer Institute; NHLBI = National Heart, Lung, and Blood Institute; NIA = National Institute on Aging; NIAID = National Institute of Allergy and Infectious Diseases; NIAMS = National Institute of Arthritis and Musculoskeletal and Skin Diseases; NICHD = National Institute of Child Health and Human Development; NIDA = National Institute on Drug Abuse; NIDDK = National Institute of Diabetes and Digestive and Kidney Diseases; NIMH = National Institute of Mental Health; NINDS = National Institute of Neurological Disorders and Stroke.
SOURCE: NIH, 2012b. Reprinted with permission from the National Institutes of Health/U.S. Department of Health and Human Services.

BOX 3-2
Selected Examples of NIH Institute Uses
of CTSA Skills and Capacities

National Cancer Institute (NCI)

- Cancer centers have benefited from CTSAs' experience in educating and mentoring investigators, community outreach, clinical facilities, and pilot project programs (Weiss, 2012).

- NCI projects and CTSAs invest in a range of shared resources, such as biostatistics and laboratory management tools and biorepositories and genomics resources. They also jointly support pilot projects, faculty and staff recruitment and training programs, clinical research infrastructure, and community-based research through practice-based research networks, mobile clinical research units, and e-health programs (Weiss, 2012).

National Institute of Allergy and Infectious Diseases (NIAID)

- NIAID Clinical Research Centers use CTSA support for research volunteer recruitment (e.g., 34 allergy and infectious disease-related studies used ResearchMatch, and 110 NIAID-related pilot projects were funded) (CTSA Central, 2011b).

National Institute of Diabetes and Digestive and Kidney Diseases (NIDDK)

- CTSAs provide support for many NIDDK-funded large clinical trials and networks. For example, most of NIDDK's liver disease consortia and the Drug-Induced Liver Injury Network have used CTSA infrastructure for follow-up activities (Germino, 2012).

The way that skills and resources available through the CTSA Program can be translated into tangible support for institute and center grants and projects is further illustrated by these more detailed examples:

- NeuroNEXT, a National Institute of Neurological Disorders and Stroke network to conduct Phase 2 clinical trials in neurological disorders of children and adults, has 25 clinical sites, 23 of which also have CTSA awards. The network is in its early phases and is collaborating with the CTSA Program whenever possible in order to connect researchers with CTSA resources; the NeuroNEXT RFA specifically asked applicants to identify how they would interact with CTSAs. A number of overlapping goals between the network and the CTSAs include the use of central institutional review board (IRB) processes and standing trial agreements across sites and early involvement of patient advocacy groups (Kaufmann, 2013).

- The University of Iowa's CTSA provides support to meet the informatics needs of a multidisciplinary team that was awarded a 5-year, $3 million grant from the National Cancer Institute to develop image analysis tools that will be used in future clinical trials to better assess patient responses to cancer treatments (NIH, 2012b).

- Three California CTSAs are collaborating with the Stanford Synchrotron Radiation Lightsource[2] to develop an automated and customizable drug discovery pipeline called "Auto-Drug," which can screen samples that could be used to develop new pharmacological treatments for a variety of diseases (NIH, 2012b; Stanford University, 2012; Tsai et al., 2012).

- The National Heart, Lung, and Blood Institute's ongoing multisite trial, the International Study of Comparative Health Effectiveness with Medical and Invasive Approaches (ISCHEMIA), used the CTSA resource IRBShare to help participating institutions share review documents and review processes on a secure web portal (Shurin, 2012).

- The National Institute on Drug Abuse used set-aside funds for three studies at CTSA sites: an examination of models to reduce disparities in clinical trials, including recruitment and retention of drug users and underrepresented populations; an experimental trial of a drug to reduce opioid overdose; and a study on how best to prevent drug abuse among Hispanic adolescents (Volkow, 2012).

The IOM committee believes that many of the challenges in clinical and translational research must be solved using systemwide approaches and that the CTSA Program is well positioned, perhaps uniquely so, to facilitate and implement those approaches. The combination of local, disease-specific resources and the more general collaborative approaches and tools developed under the CTSA Program strengthen the potential contribution CTSAs can make when partnered with projects funded by NIH institutes and centers. In addition, these types of partnerships and

---

[2]Stanford Synchrotron Radiation Lightsource is a research tool that uses extremely bright X-rays to study compounds and other samples at atomic and molecular levels (Stanford University, 2013).

collaborations provide opportunities to optimize available resources and to increase efficiency and cost-effectiveness. Collaborative efforts would go a long way toward "dissolving the artificial barriers that inevitably spring up in any large organization," a benefit envisioned at the time of the program's launch (Zerhouni, 2005, p. 1622). In a sense, this represents a scaling up of the program sites' success at building academic homes for clinical and translational research, reducing intradepartmental boundaries to collaboration, and developing regional collaborations (Briggs and Austin, 2012).

Partnerships with Health Care Providers, Health Care Systems, and Practice-Based Research Networks

Beginning in 2007, the IOM, through its Roundtable on Evidence-Based Medicine (now the Roundtable on Value & Science-Driven Health Care), has examined a broad range of topics related to reengineering clinical research and health care delivery so as to support a continuously learning health care system (see Chapter 2) (IOM, 2007, 2013b). Built on the foundation of a strong digital infrastructure, innovative health care models, research on practice, and aligned incentives, the learning health care system offers the promise of more efficient and effective clinical care.

The work of CTSAs can bear directly on the nation's ability to achieve a learning health care system through collaborations that strengthen ties between the realms of practice and research. Among the strongest candidates for these types of CTSA collaborations are practice-based research networks (PBRNs) and the HMO Research Network (HMORN).

PBRNs are "groups of primary care clinicians and practices working together to answer community-based health care questions and translate research findings into practice" (AHRQ, 2012). As of 2011, almost 13,000 primary care practices (providing care to approximately 47.5 million people) were involved in PBRNs, and just over half of them (52 percent) were affiliated with CTSAs (Peterson et al., 2012). Several surveys of the relationship between CTSAs and PBRNs have found disappointingly low levels of community engagement and collaboration. In a 2008 survey, PBRN directors noted that the value of CTSAs to PBRNs included funding, aid with IRB processes, biostatistics, training, and consultation. In return, PBRNs were in a position to help CTSAs move their research into community settings and improve connections between CTSA home institutions and the community (Fagnan et al., 2010). Nevertheless, these relationships were not without challenges. For example, "CTSA leaders often sought PBRNs as study recruiting sites . . . but they seemed less aware of the need for cultivating ongoing relationships and the importance of engaging practitioners in the support and development of study protocols" (Fagnan et al., 2010, p. 482).

In 2011, PBRNs registering with the AHRQ's National PBRN Resource Center noted that having a relationship with a CTSA made no significant difference in PBRN research opportunities or capacity (Peterson et al., 2012). The researchers reported that "although 63 registered PBRNs (52 percent) reported a formal affiliation with a CTSA, in 2011 these PBRNs conducted the same number of studies as PBRNs not affiliated with a CTSA" (Peterson et al., 2012, p. 568). Calmbach and colleagues (2012) characterized the relationship between CTSAs and PBRNs as "a process that still is developing" (p. 572). While partnerships with CTSAs may be helpful in increasing support for PBRNs and raising their visibility, these partnerships also "could be detrimental if the university tries to impose a top-down research agenda onto already busy primary care physicians" (Calmbach et al., 2012, p. 572). Further, the institutions may not fully appreciate the costs to the physicians' practices of participation in CTSA projects.

As noted in these articles, support for the concept of collaboration between the academic researchers and clinicians working in the community remains strong despite the time and effort involved in forging strong relationships and the difficulties noted. The development of electronic health records and their use as part of a learning health care system, as well as the work of the Patient-Centered Outcomes Research Institute, may enable and motivate closer working relationships between researchers and clinicians in the future. The CTSA Program offers a venue and mechanisms for these types of partnerships, which are critical to the future of translational sciences.

Another potential source of clinician partnerships is offered by the HMORN, a network of 18 U.S. health care delivery organizations with recognized research departments or institutes that also have a defined patient population (HMO Research Network, 2013). Input to the IOM committee from the HMORN Governing Board indicated that 14 HMORN sites have established relationships with local CTSAs, and 1 HMORN site has two such relationships. One site has discontinued its CTSA relationship

(Steiner, 2013). Suggestions from HMORN board members for improved collaborations included the following:

- development of partnerships that are aligned by purpose and values;
- expanded pilot funding for community-based investigators;
- expanded bidirectional training opportunities; and
- ongoing education for members of academic leadership about the importance of research related to defined populations and then translating findings into community-based delivery systems (Steiner, 2013).

HMORN board members made several suggestions for ways in which the CTSA Program could become a more effective incubator for innovation. These suggestions included more coordinated outreach by CTSA-HMORN partners to underserved populations; broader use of supplemental funds to support HMORN dissemination of "translatable" research findings; strategic application of pilot funds to codevelop innovations; and increased incentives for community-based clinical trials (Steiner, 2013). HMORN board members suggested that the NIH-initiated Health Care Systems Research Collaboratory may be an example of how collaborative work between CTSAs and HMORN could work in the future.[3]

Partnerships with Industry

As with community-based clinician involvement, partnerships with industry have been viewed as essential components of the CTSA Program from the beginning. In a 2010 meeting organized by the NIH, senior industry executives formally met with CTSA awardee scientists for the first time to discuss ways to advance both groups' goals. Although general consensus exists about the desirability of moving useful innovations quickly and safely into clinical care, how to achieve this goal is much less obvious (Fine, 2012; Wadman, 2010).

Among the obstacles to greater CTSA-industry partnerships are intellectual property constraints and concerns about conflicts of interest.

---

[3]The Health Care Systems Research Collaboratory, housed at Duke University, is a coordinating center for a set of pragmatic randomized trials involving HMORN sites. The center is currently developing and disseminating collaborative research tools to the investigator community, including the NIH Distributed Research Network (Steiner, 2013).

"We are not able to work effectively together because of the perception and reality of conflict of interest," one industry participant said (Wadman, 2010, p. 256), although some instances were cited in which these concerns have been overcome. One initiative described at the conference is Eli Lilly and Company's not-for-profit tuberculosis drug consortium,[4] which links academic investigators to expertise and tools donated by Eli Lilly, Merck, private foundations, the National Institute of Allergy and Infectious Diseases, and the nonprofit Infectious Disease Research Institute (NIAID, 2012). Another is Merck's new Calibr (California Institute for Biomedical Research) initiative, a nonprofit organization intended to speed the development of innovative new medicines (Fine, 2012). Similarly, the Indiana Clinical and Translational Science Institute formed a partnership with Veeda Clinical Research and Eli Lilly to develop a shared research facility for first-in-human studies and other early phase studies (NIH, 2012b).

At the IOM committee's December 2012 meeting, Jacqueline Fine of Merck Research Laboratories spoke specifically about collaborative opportunities in early phases of translational research (Fine, 2012). She pointed out that, from industry's point of view, successful translation is not achieved until an innovation becomes part of the standard of care. The activities that will facilitate this process, including regulatory approval and other favorable policy actions, should be thought about at the front end of a project. It is not clear to industry leaders that academic researchers, accustomed to nondirected discovery, are sufficiently focused on those end-of-the-process considerations (Fine, 2012). Successful partnerships in this arena will require identification of shared goals and an understanding of the roles and value that each of the partners brings to the table.

The CTSA Program provides a unique venue to build strategic partnerships and collaborations between academia and private-sector partners, including pharmaceutical and biotech companies and companies involved in the development of medical devices, technologies, and diagnostics. These partnerships and collaborations will be imperative to realizing the program's streamlined mission. Characteristics that may facilitate effective industry-CTSA relationships include a simple and transparent interface for partnering including shared strategies and priorities, a clear mission for CTSAs and their multisite collaboratives, the willing-

---

[4]See http://www.tbdrugdiscovery.org (accessed March 26, 2013).

ness of individual CTSAs or CTSA groups to align their focus with that of an industry partner, and an ethical and transparent relationship.

The CTSA Program needs to explore and implement new approaches for collaboration with industry that foster the translation of research into products while remaining within legal and regulatory boundaries. In addition, the CTSA Program can serve as a leader in promoting innovation, entrepreneurship, and cultural changes; developing and testing new approaches for managing conflict of interest and intellectual property; and engaging the Food and Drug Administration and other regulators in collaborations. As these partnerships are established and grow, it will be important for NCATS and the CTSAs to share and implement best practices.

Opportunities and Next Steps

Collaborations across and among researchers and research networks are core to building an integrated network that supports the work of clinical and translational science. Because the CTSA Program is a facilitator and accelerator of this research, NCATS, the CTSA Program, and individual CTSA sites need to ensure that they are working to initiate, nurture, and strengthen collaborations across CTSA institutions, with NIH institutes and centers, with private- and public-sector research institutions and networks, and with community stakeholders. With their core focus on strengthening the infrastructure of clinical and translational research, CTSAs are ideal partners for all these entities.

Mutually beneficial collaborations take time, energy, and initiative to build and sustain. All sides need to find value in the partnership, and all need to work to maintain and further shared goals. Sufficient incentives for collaboration may be inherent in the partnering organizations' ongoing priorities, but in many cases, external incentives may be needed in order to provide the impetus to collaborate.

The IOM committee urges NCATS to establish a CTSA innovations fund that would provide incentives for creating new collaborations and supporting collaborative pilot studies or resource-sharing initiatives. For example, such projects might require the collaboration of multiple CTSAs, might jointly involve CTSAs and PBRNs or other research networks, or might engage groups of CTSAs and NIH institutes or centers. These collaborative projects might also involve new industry or community partners, other government agencies (e.g., the AHRQ, Food and Drug Administration, Department of Veterans Affairs, or public and private research entities. The fund could be used to support collaborative initiatives to develop novel strategies for implementation research that would be tested in multiple locations. This fund could be created through a set-aside mechanism within the CTSA Program that provides flexible funding to foster collaborative efforts that are pioneering and have great potential to accelerate clinical and translational research. Projects associated with this fund should include clear metrics and evaluation measures.

INDIVIDUAL CTSAs

The NIH developed the CTSA Program in order to increase the speed and efficiency with which new ideas and technologies would move from the research laboratory into clinical and community practice. Accomplishing this objective has required strengthening many research activities in academic health centers (and other institutions), such as biomedical informatics and training for researchers, as well as a focused effort to find efficient and effective ways to share resources and develop common tools, databases, and research processes, all with the ultimate goal of improving human health. Building an active and productive CTSA at an academic health center or other institution often involves not only the funds from the CTSA cooperative agreement but also substantial financial and staff commitments from the institution; although institutional cost sharing is not required. The committee could not identify any data to quantify these institutional contributions but heard testimony from many individuals about the depth of efforts and the commitment to the CTSA Program from top leaders at health research institutions across the nation.

In its first 7 years, the CTSA Program has done much to develop and nurture the CTSA sites as academic homes for clinical and translational research with an emphasis on training researchers, providing shared resources, streamlining and improving clinical research management, and developing community and research partnerships. Zerhouni (2005) defined an academic home as a place that provides intellectual and physical resources for original clinical and translational science. He envisioned CTSAs as creating "environments that over time provide the theoretical underpinnings of the discipline, provide much needed education programs, contribute to the growth of well structured and well recognized career pathways, and provide a research environment more nimble, conducive to and responsive to the demands of modern translational and clinical research" (Zerhouni, 2005, p. 1622). Progress has been made in creating these academic homes. The challenges ahead will be to capital-ize on these efforts and refocus the program so that it becomes a network that is responsive, nimble, and innovative in accelerating clinical and translational research.

The early funding announcements for the CTSA Program identified a set of key functions that evolved over time, some of which became a re-quired part of the program. Some of the key functions were as follows:

- Development of novel clinical and translational methodologies
- Research education, training, and career development
- Pilot and collaborative translational and clinical studies
- Biomedical informatics
- Design, biostatistics, and clinical research ethics
- Regulatory knowledge and support
- Clinical research resources and facilities
- Community engagement
- Evaluation
- Translational technologies and resources (NIH, 2005, 2009).

In its most recent CTSA funding announcement, the NIH changed the criteria so that applicants were given greater flexibility to build on the strengths of their home institutions in specific phases of clinical and translational research (T0–T4) or in a specific area of research (e.g., child health research) (NCATS, 2012b; NIH, 2012c).

The 61 CTSA sites provide a wide array of training and research re-sources to help researchers identify promising therapeutics and interven-tions and move them forward as rapidly as feasible, as discussed in Chapter 1. These resources often require large institutional investments in purchasing equipment and instruments, renovating space, and provid-ing at least partial support for staff. Despite the availability of these re-sources, researchers in some institutions have reported that they were unaware of the core resources or found them too expensive or cumber-some to use (Curley, 2013; Raue et al., 2011). A central database cata-loging CTSA resources has been developed (CTSA Central, 2013b), but questions regarding the cost of using the resources and visibility contin-ue, according to testimony received by the IOM committee from a num-ber of involved individuals.

CTSAs have worked to facilitate and simplify clinical research man-agement through the use of project managers or navigators and other mechanisms and tools. For example, CTSA sites are attempting to ensure efficient protocol development processes and limit required review steps to those that actually add value to the final research protocol. In a partial inventory of the process improvements that had been achieved, as of 2010, 15 sites reported they had developed process maps, and at least 20 reported improvements that, in some cases, reduced processing times by more than 30 percent. Some of these improvements resulted from streamlining IRB approvals (Rosenblum and Alving, 2011).

Variation in the activities of individual CTSAs has grown up across the program due in part to the range of CTSA site funding (from $4 million to $23 million in fiscal year [FY] 2012) (Briggs and Austin, 2012) and in part to differences in home institution governance structures, management styles, and the areas of focus and depth in research portfolios (Rosenblum and Alving, 2011). Although the CTSA Program is disease agnostic in its overall resources and approach, the individual CTSA sites may facilitate research on specific conditions, and their home institutions may be research leaders in those areas. Thus the individual CTSAs and the program as a whole provide great potential to augment and facilitate the disease-specific work of NIH institutes and centers, as well as that of their home institutions (see Box 3-3). The CTSA Program supports disease-specific research in a variety of ways, which may include funding, research tools and facilities, expert consultation, research participant recruitment, and other research resources and support mechanisms described in Chapter 1. In its assessment of the CTSA Program, the committee identified numerous examples of disease-specific research connected to the Program. The types of CTSA resources that were used to support the research were rarely identified or described, however.

BOX 3-3
Examples of Disease-Specific Research Aided by CTSA Resources

Cancer: An international team of researchers led by Weill Cornell Medical College investigators identified two inherited gene deletions that more than triple the risk of aggressive prostate cancer (Demichelisa et al., 2012; Woods, 2012).

Heart disease: Using financial support and an information network provided by Harvard's CTSA, investigators at Beth Israel Deaconess Medical Center used a mouse model to develop molecular evidence that helps explain why preeclampsia and multiple gestation are risk factors for peripartum cardiomyopathy, a sometimes fatal condition that develops in 1 in 3,000 pregnant women with no known heart disease history (Patten et al., 2012; Prescott, 2012).

Lung disease: Leading a 175-person research team in 13 sites in Japan, Canada, and the United States, with partial CTSA funding, University of Cincinnati researchers identified a treatment for a rare, severe lung disease (lymphangioleiomyomatosis) that affects women in their childbearing years (McCormack et al., 2011; Pence, 2012)

Muscular dystrophy: Using a national database developed by the University of Rochester Medical Center, researchers explored the impact of symptoms on the lives of patients with muscular dystrophy and found that those symptoms affecting daily life (e.g., fatigue, limited mobility) are more important to patients than those most commonly associated with muscular dystrophy (e.g., myotonia). Study results are being used to improve patient outcome measures and could be used to target future treatment (Heatwole et al., 2012; Michaud, 2012).

Stroke: Physicians at Barnes-Jewish Hospital used partial funding through Washington University in St. Louis's CTSA to reduce the average time between a stroke patient's arrival and treatment from 58 to 37 minutes by eliminating inefficient steps in the care process. Rapid administration of anticlotting medication is key to preventing brain damage from stroke (Purdy, 2012).

Opportunities and Next Steps

Individual CTSAs have made progress in establishing academic homes for clinical and translational research. The challenge for CTSA 2.0 will be to create a national network of institutions that are engaged in accelerating clinical and translational science. In its assessment of the program, the IOM committee heard many questions from stakeholders about the optimal number of individual CTSAs. The committee did not choose to specify an ideal number, but rather believes that over time the number could change as strategic goals and priorities are set and as determinations are made about future program directions. The focus should not be on the absolute number of CTSAs but on whether the CTSAs are achieving progress as measured by defined goals and priorities.

As described in Chapter 1, individual CTSAs, the CTSA Program, and NCATS need to continually push to identify effective therapeutics and interventions and move them to the individuals and populations that could benefit from them. The IOM committee realizes that this major undertaking will move forward in incremental steps as well as major leaps. For individual CTSAs, the challenge will be to keep their home institutions engaged and active while reaching out to develop the collaborations with other CTSAs, research networks, industry, and community stakeholders. Effective clinical and translational research requires creativity and innovation that could be ignited by collaboration across disciplines and beyond the biomedical and health sciences. In order to tackle the most complex and pressing health challenges, CTSAs should attempt to create partnerships with schools of business, law, engineering, nursing, public health, and communications, as well as with relevant academic departments, such as anthropology and psychology.

The IOM committee supports the recent change to the CTSA RFA that allows greater flexibility for individual CTSA sites to focus on the strengths of their institutions. Recognizing that some CTSAs may excel in early discovery science, others in later development research, and others in implementation of findings in the community, it will still be critically important for NCATS to ensure that the CTSA Program, as a whole, covers the full spectrum of clinical and translational research. Further, sites should retain their emphasis on community engagement in order to ensure participation and breadth of input by community practitioners, patients, and other stakeholders (see Chapter 4).

The IOM committee urges NCATS and CTSAs to continue to foster integrated research communities of CTSAs with common interests and expertise, to share infrastructure further, to work on common projects, and to strengthen collaborations. Individual CTSAs are encouraged to identify and implement efficient and cost-effective ways to provide access to core facilities and resources. Further efforts are needed to promote awareness of their many resources, training, and services and to reduce their costs.

EVALUATION

Stakeholders, including research funders, the public, and Congress, increasingly demand evidence of returns on investments in the health research enterprise, such as advances in clinical practice and increases in the availability of new therapeutics and interventions (Austin, 2013; Reed et al., 2012; Shuster, 2012). Evaluation can be an incentive or catalyst for positive change and improved outcomes and is necessary for accountability, transparency, informed decision making, and communication about outcomes and the value of an investment.[5] In a multifaceted and complex effort such as the CTSA Program, evaluation is a formidable undertaking, but one that is vital to ensuring accountability and planning for future directions. Over the life of the CTSA Program, the NIH has recognized the importance of evaluation by building it into the requirements for the first set of CTSA awards, maintaining the requirement for each of the subsequent CTSA awards, and initiating an external evaluation process that assessed the program as a whole, as described below.

Evaluating Individual CTSAs

As part of the application process for a CTSA award, applicants are required to have a plan in place to

- monitor the use, quality, and costs associated with the programs, resources, and services that are provided;
- assess data and modify programs, resources, and services as necessary in order to better meet the needs of researchers, increase quality and efficiency, and reduce costs; and
- track and assess innovative methods and practices related to the structure, aggregation, and provision of services, programs, and resources (NIH, 2012c).

The recent RFA also requests "a full description of tracking processes, metrics, and milestones proposed to ensure ongoing assessment and timely adjustment of activities of the CTSA" (NIH, 2012c). Individual CTSA evaluation plans correspond to the varying needs and capacities of an individual CTSA's structure, available funding, and programs and activities supported. This diversity makes cross-CTSA evaluation a challenge that may become even more difficult as individual CTSAs are given more latitude to specialize. However, some salient summative measures are necessary in order to establish program accountability and to demonstrate its progress and value as a whole. Cross-CTSA evaluation

---

[5]The definition of "evaluation" used for this report is from Patton's work on utilization-focused evaluation: "Program evaluation is the systemic collection of information about the activities, characteristics, and results of programs to make judgments about the program, improve or further develop program effectiveness, inform decisions about future programming, and/or increase understanding" (Patton, 2008).

will require high-level common metrics and measures that can be applied consistently at all sites.

Self-Evaluations of the Individual CTSAs

Each CTSA site conducts internal assessments of its own activities, processes, and performance. Individual CTSAs report a median of three members on their evaluation teams representing 1.3 full-time equivalents (FTEs) on average. Approximately three-quarters of evaluation teams, however, report significant assistance from other staff in evaluation efforts, which may not be captured in the FTEs reported (Alexander et al., 2013). Sites often use mixed-methods approaches that may include quantitative data collection, satisfaction surveys, social network analysis, focus groups, interviews, and case studies. Many use a systems approach that assesses programmatic components individually and collectively (Alexander et al., 2013; Rubio et al., 2012).

The 2012 National CTSA Evaluators Survey[6] recognized robust evaluation efforts across the program cumulatively, but also identified significant heterogeneity in strategies and methods being employed at individual CTSAs. The authors concluded that the heterogeneity represents both a strength, in terms of diversity and flexibility, and a challenge with regard to obtaining standardized information (Alexander et al., 2013). The IOM committee noted variability in publicly available information on the individual CTSAs' evaluation efforts and overall accomplishments—for example, some CTSAs post information about their broad evaluation plans on their websites,[7] and some include impact information.[8] However, descriptions of these evaluation processes, metrics, and outcomes are not consistently available for public information.

Although flexibility in the evaluation approaches and processes of the individual CTSAs is appropriate given their variation in size, structure, and focus, some level of standardization is also needed. The National CTSA Evaluators Survey highlighted challenges related to a lack

---

[6]For the last 3 years, the Shared Resources Working Group of the Evaluation Key Function Committee (described below) has used the National CTSA Evaluators Survey to assess the evaluation management and methods being applied across the individual CTSAs and to identify emerging challenges and new evaluation tools in use, such as dashboard technologies (Alexander et al., 2013; Rubio et al., 2012).

[7]See, for example, http://casemed.case.edu/ctsc/cores/evaluation.cfm; http://dccweb2.bumc.bu.edu/wordpress/index.php/programs/program-tracking-and-evaluation (accessed April 10, 2013).

[8]See, for example, http://ctsi.ucsf.edu/impact (accessed April 10, 2013).

of common metrics, clear definitions, and guidance from funders (Alexander et al., 2013). Overcoming these obstacles needs to be a priority in order to implement effective evaluation strategies that will ensure sufficient consistency and establish accountability.

Fostering Best Practices

In the early phases of the CTSA Program, the Evaluation Key Function Committee was established to provide "a forum for institutions to exchange information about their evaluation approaches, challenges, and progress" (CTSA Central, 2013f). This key function committee and its working groups are making strides to foster best practices and improve evaluations being conducted at the individual CTSA level. Every other month the committee produces a newsletter and hosts a cohort call during which two CTSAs present evaluation strategies and challenges. Members of the key function committee have found these presentations valuable for sharing best practices and identifying common challenges (and possible solutions) encountered in the sites' self-evaluation processes (personal communication, D. Rubio, University of Pittsburgh, March 15, 2013).

The Evaluation Key Function Committee is attempting to develop common metrics in specific areas that could be used as benchmarks for individual CTSAs and the CTSA Program as a whole. It is currently working across the consortium committees to develop, test, and implement common metrics related to clinical research processes and outcomes. While in the early stages of development, this effort is focusing on 15 metrics in areas such as clinical research processes, careers, services, economic return, collaboration, and products (Rubio, 2013).

The committee has advised other key function committees on the development of common metrics also. For example, it worked with the Biostatistics, Epidemiology, and Research Design Key Function Committee to develop consensus on 56 performance items related to collaboration, use of existing methods, and discovery of new methods (Rubio et al., 2011a); it consulted with the Community Engagement Key Function Committee in developing the evaluation section of *Principles of Community Engagement* and with the Education and Career Development Key Function Committee to develop common metrics for measuring career success (Lee et al., 2012; Rubio et al., 2011b, 2012; Task Force on the Principles of Community Engagement, 2011).

Finally, the evaluation committee's National Evaluation Liaison Working Group consulted with the American Evaluation Association to propose an evaluation framework for the CTSA Program (Rubio et al., 2012). The framework was developed to provide recommendations to NCATS and other program stakeholders on how the program could be evaluated effectively, given its complexity. The recommendations focus on a range of areas that include scope of evaluation, structure and organization, funding, methodology, utilization, policy, and capacity (CTSA Evaluation Key Function Committee, 2012). This framework has the potential to serve as a valuable resource for NCATS as it considers its next steps in implementing the CTSA Program and in identifying approaches to evaluating individual CTSAs and the program as a whole.

NCATS's Role in Evaluating Individual CTSAs

As part of their award obligations, CTSA sites must submit annual progress reports to NCATS, describing their accomplishments, milestones, challenges, and the barriers affecting their work. The Office of Management and Budget is requiring that the progress report format be updated and standardized across agencies; the new format will capture information on accomplishments, products, participants, impact, changes, special reporting requirements, and budget (NIH, 2012a). The IOM committee understands, however, that the new format will reduce flexibility in the types of specific information that NCATS can request as part of the reporting process (personal communication, E. Collier, NCATS, March 20, 2013).

Despite a statement in the recent RFA that "the NIH is committed to transparency in the CTSA Program to ensure the program is delivering on its mission" (NIH, 2012c), no parts of the sites' annual progress reports are publicly available (nor were they available to the committee). In addition, the progress reports are not currently used for evaluation purposes, according to NCATS staff (Parsons, 2013). The IOM committee cannot say whether these required progress reports are the most appropriate way to evaluate the individual CTSAs or the program or to communicate annual progress, not having inspected them. Nevertheless, the committee strongly believes that, given the size of this investment, there must be a mechanism in place that requires *all* of the individual CTSAs to regularly and publicly report on defined metrics, milestones, and accomplishments. From the IOM committee's perspective, this lack of public information thwarts the need to ensure transparency and accountability.

During the December 2012 IOM committee workshop, NCATS staff reported that the NIH's current primary evaluation mechanism for CTSA sites is the peer-review process associated with renewal applications for the cooperative agreements (Briggs, 2012). The recent RFA provided an extensive list of review criteria that will be used to assess these applications; however, it is unclear how NCATS evaluates the CTSAs during the 5-year award cycle and what mechanisms are in place for midterm assessments or any necessary corrective actions. The committee urges NCATS to assert leadership in improving transparency in reporting of metrics, milestones, and accomplishments at the individual CTSA level and to ensure that sufficient accountability monitoring is in place through a set of common metrics that reflect the program's mission and strategic goals.

Evaluating the CTSA Program

Various aspects of the CTSA Program have been evaluated. External evaluations by Westat provided quantitative and qualitative baseline measures for the program. That 3-year evaluation used site visits to assess training and education, resource utilization, publications, and the overall progress of individual CTSAs (see Box 3-4). Westat's final

---

BOX 3-4
Evaluations of the CTSA Program

Report on Field Visits to the CTSAs (Westat, 2011): Westat conducted site visits at 9 CTSA institutions with interviews of 369 individuals in various positions. Despite variation across the sites, Westat concluded that the CTSAs are making progress on meeting program goals related to building infrastructure, training and education, and translation of research findings into practice. Participating interviewees across the sites indicated that CTSA support had enabled progress in clinical and translational research that would not have been made otherwise. The report points out that at the time of these interviews, the program was still in its early stages and notes that many aspects of the program were still evolving, especially those related to building collaborations.

Findings from the CTSA National Evaluation Education and Training Study (Miyaoka et al., 2011): Westat surveyed 553 CTSA-supported scholars and trainees and 665 mentors and found that both groups were very positive in their review of the education and training components of the CTSA program. Areas identified for improvement included increasing the ethnic diversity of mentors, scholars, and trainees; expanding training in team science and technology transfer; and dedicating more resources to the online learning and career planning components of the program.

Findings from the CTSA National Evaluation Utilization Study (Raue et al., 2011): Westat conducted a survey of 302 users of CTSA resources and 537 nonusers, all of whom worked for one of the initial 46 CTSA sites that were established between 2006 and 2009. A large majority of nonusers (80 percent) conducted nonclinical research, and 48 percent indicated they did not need additional resources. The evaluators highlighted the wide range of research resources available and found that 79 percent of the users were satisfied with those resources. However, the report cited a lack of awareness and confusion about the program and its resources and noted a need for increased visibility and communication.

Final Report on CTSA-Supported Publications: 2006 to 2011 (Steketee et al., 2012): Westat analyzed the CTSA sites' annual progress reports and online journal databases and found 17,038 publications identified as supported by CTSA resources. Evaluators indicated that publications per CTSA institution increased every year it had CTSA funding and found a growing number of publications that involved collaboration between more than one CTSA. The report identified a need for improvements in standardization in reporting CTSA-supported publications; more than 2,800 publications that cited CTSA support were not included in awardee annual progress reports, and 85 percent of publications listed in the annual reports did not cite CTSA funding.

The CTSA National Evaluation Phase 1 Final Report (Frechtling et al., 2012): This report concluded that the CTSA Program is enabling a new research infrastructure and encouraging the adoption of new practices that have the potential to streamline the clinical and translational research process. Westat recommended that, going forward, the program should support institutional pilot programs, increase awareness of the program and available resources, expand education and training opportunities, streamline the CTSA Consortium, increase incentives for collaboration and partnership, and conduct long-term evaluations.

summary report concluded that "the CTSA program is making important strides toward encouraging and enhancing a new kind of medical research infrastructure and re-engineering the scientific research process" (Frechtling et al., 2012, p. vii). In addition, the OIG evaluated the administration of the CTSA Program under the NCRR (discussed earlier in the chapter) (OIG, 2011).

Despite these previous efforts and the obvious commitment to evaluation at the CTSA site level, the committee is not aware of future plans to evaluate the overall program. The IOM committee believes that a formal, programwide evaluation process should be undertaken to measure progress toward NCATS's vision for CTSA 2.0. Elements that could be considered in developing metrics have been identified by NCATS staff (Briggs and Austin, 2012) and by the IOM committee and include the extent to which program awardees are facilitating clinical studies, with an emphasis on multisite studies; advancing the translation of research findings into therapeutics, diagnostics, and preventive interventions; developing innovative research methods; promoting community engagement; training and educating the next generation of clinical and translational researchers; protecting human subjects and reducing delays in clinical trials; developing informatics standards; and promoting data resources and research tools.

In addition to the evaluations described, additional reporting mechanisms document and communicate the accomplishments of CTSA sites and the CTSA Consortium. For example, the CTSA Consortium committees produce an annual report recounting the activities and achievements of each committee, working group, and task force. These reports detail a range of activities, from small-scale accomplishments, such as establishing committee-specific e-mail addresses, to larger efforts, such as developing a catalog of unique T1 resources available through the program (CTSA Central, 2011a). The CTSA Consortium compiled an extensive list of activities that demonstrates the breadth and capabilities of the program for the NIH CTSA/NCATS Integration Working Group (Katz et al., 2011; Pulley, 2013).

In addition, the NIH has produced two progress reports that cover accomplishments of individual CTSAs and the CTSA Consortium from 2006 to 2008 and 2009 to 2011 (NCRR, 2009; NIH, 2012b). The most recent report highlights specific examples of program accomplishments in six key areas: accelerating discoveries, improving clinical research efficiency, training the next generation of investigators, fostering collaboration and partnerships, enhancing the health of communities and the nation, and developing resources and networking for sharing data. Just as some individual CTSAs feature information on achievements on their websites, the NCATS website has a page that includes stories about successes attributed to the CTSA Program and other NCATS-supported programs (NCATS, 2013d).

These mechanisms, although not part of a formal evaluation process, are important for communicating the value of the program. They could be modified to include specific detail on how CTSAs contributed to particular accomplishments or which program resources were used to achieve them. They also could be used to report results of a more formalized evaluation process. The NIH and NCATS should report on any programwide evaluation findings in pursuit of transparency, and as mentioned previously, there should be a mechanism in place for individual CTSAs to report regularly on defined metrics, milestones, and accomplishments.

Opportunities and Next Steps

The IOM committee believes that a set of clearly defined, measurable strategic goals is the starting point for shaping the CTSA Program's future. These measurable goals should serve as a foundation for developing high-level common metrics and measures that could be applied and reported consistently to demonstrate progress. At this point, NCATS's plans for evaluating individual CTSA sites and the CTSA Program as a whole are unclear. Progress is being made at the individual CTSA level in terms of self-evaluation, but the current lack of transparency in reporting and lack of high-level common metrics are barriers to overall program accountability.

Developing common metrics that can be implemented across the CTSAs will be a formidable challenge that will require input and cooperation from all the CTSAs. The complexity of the CTSA Program may also require the application of innovative metrics that go beyond standard academic benchmarks of publications and number of grants awarded.

The ultimate goal of clinical and translational research, and therefore the ultimate goal of the CTSA Program, is to improve human health. Although it would be ideal to evaluate the CTSA Program's impact on clinical care and public health, currently this is neither feasible nor realistic given the numerous driving forces that shape the research enterprise (see Chapter 2) and the multitude of factors that affect health outcomes. In addition, there are multiple direct and indirect ways in which the CTSA Program contributes to research infrastructure and resources, collaborations, cultural changes, training, and community engagement that influence clinical and translational research but cannot be easily identified or measured. Despite these and other such challenges, the CTSA Program can be a leader in developing evaluation methodologies and metrics that could provide more real-time assessments of progress in advancing clinical and translational research, overcoming research barriers, fulfilling the program's mission and strategic goals, and, whenever possible, changing clinical care and improving public health.

COMMUNICATIONS

A common underlying theme to establishing leadership and account-ability is effective communication. "The effective communication of sci-entific results and viewpoints to the public is an important responsibility of the scientific community. This is particularly so for science that has been publicly funded" (ICSU CFRS, 2010, p. 1). In this report, the IOM committee takes a broad perspective on the role of communications. It does not mean only an occasional news release or printed report, but ra-ther the full array of activities and methods of communication undertak-en to attract partners, achieve transparency and accountability, promote public support and understanding of findings, and ensure that findings are acted on, whether they relate to advances affecting clinical care or ways to improve the working of the scientific enterprise. Communication in this global sense is fundamental to clinical and translational research. It is likewise fundamental to conveying and achieving the value added from the CTSA Program.

In part, the need for a robust and diverse communications effort has been anticipated through the creation of two entities: the Communica-tions Key Function Committee and the CTSA Consortium Coordinating Center. The key function committee provides the opportunity for CTSA and NIH information officers and staff "to share local and national CTSA communications best practices, activities and experiences; and to identify and generate ideas to address CTSA communications opportuni-ties and challenges" (CTSA Central, 2013e). The committee's *Year in Review* report highlights best practices from individual CTSAs in their use of a range of media, including social media, to highlight their work and attempt to educate the public generally about clinical and transla-tional research (CTSA Central, 2013c).

When the CTSA Consortium Coordinating Center was established in November 2011, its role explicitly included enhancing communications through organizing networking resources and enabling outreach and dis-semination of tools. Although some overlap may exist in mission be-tween the Coordinating Center and the key function committee, the latter's efforts appear more heavily focused on media dissemination, whereas the Coordinating Center's role is more directed to providing technical assistance and facilitating communication within the program. To the extent that the Communications Key Function Committee and Coordinating Center, as they evolve, cannot take on all of the communica-tions roles that might be desired, this structure might need reassessment by

NCATS. Further, a CTSA Program strategic communications plan is needed to fully implement this role.

Around the world, scientific communication efforts are slowly moving away from a strictly dissemination-based approach to a more participatory and collaborative one, as "the [Public Understanding of Science] 'paradigm of science dissemination' has been partially translated into what could be termed a 'paradigm of dialogue and participation' or Public Engagement with Science" (Felt et al., 2007, p. 55). This paradigm shift will require ongoing commitment and leadership from within the research enterprise. Signs of progress are evident at the NIH and, specifically, with the CTSA Program, wherein community engagement has been a strong part of the program from its inception. Community engagement provides a platform for collaborative dialogue and participation and encourages development of new strategies for scientific communication. Although scientists in general have resisted a more active role in communications, in part because they have not been trained for it and most likely see it as time-consuming with unclear benefit, "the lack of [professional] reward is a bigger issue" (Palmer and Schibeci, 2012, p. 12). NCATS is in a position to ameliorate this problem by, for example, including strength of communications and of community partnerships among its criteria to assess the quality of CTSA research efforts.

Both general oversight and various high-level communications activities—for example, with federal policy makers—are most appropriate for NCATS to carry out. Other, more program-specific communications activities and technical assistance might be appropriate at an intermediate level, such as by the Coordinating Center or through the communications committee. Finally, some communication activities are most effectively carried out by individual CTSA sites and projects. Box 3-5 provides examples of the opportunities at each of these levels.

BOX 3-5
Communications Opportunities Within the CTSA Program

At the broad NCATS level,

- Communicate the CTSA Program's mission and goals clearly and consistently.

- Ensure that NIH institute and center leadership know about the CTSA Program, the opportunities it offers to add value to their research efforts, and how to connect with and use it.

- Ensure that CTSA PIs and researchers appreciate the importance that NCATS places on their ability to clearly articulate the goals of their research and findings for various audiences, including community partners, and reward teams that do so effectively.

- Coordinate efforts where NCATS leverage may be needed to achieve institutional, governmental, or legislative policy changes, particularly with respect to the barriers to multi-institutional research projects (e.g., uncoordinated reviews, multiple IRB filings, and so on).

- Use what is learned from the individual CTSAs to distill best research practices that might be deployed across the nation's biomedical research enterprise and disseminate the best practices in ways that encourage their adoption.

- Maintain essential transparency and accountability through a system of reporting on both program implementation and results (IOM, 2009).

- Provide funding for professional communications staff within the Coordinating Center.

At an intermediate level (e.g., the CTSA Coordinating Center or communications-focused committee),

- Provide consultation and support for individual CTSAs and projects in their website development, media outreach, and social media strategies.

- Coordinate with other key committees as well as CTSA leadership and NCATS on media-related topics and opportunities.

- Train site representatives on effective communication with the media and public.

- Identify and share communications best practices from the sites, as with the 2011-2012 *Year in Review* report (CTSA Central, 2013c) and develop tools to simplify site adoption of these best practices.

- Provide technical assistance to sites in identifying potential audiences and communications partners (e.g., community and industry).

- Continue promotion of the specific tools and databases that sites have developed and encourage their wider adoption (at present, the Coordinating Center's website includes a listing of shareable informatics tools, and it conducts monthly webinars on how to use these tools).

- Work with sites to develop novel dissemination strategies aimed at achieving impact and sharing their findings (examples of impact would be a policy change, a clinical practice change, or an improvement in public understanding).

- Continue efforts to collect "success stories" from site efforts and developing strategies to deploy them effectively.

- Provide researchers, especially new researchers, training on appropriate communication strategies and preparing journal articles for publication.

At the individual CTSA level,

- Promote and disseminate intra-institutional communications about specific projects to maximize sharing of technical, information, and human resources within the CTSA institution and its collaborators.
- Ensure broad communication of available tools and resources across researchers within the home institution.
- Include in their teams a person with appropriate skills and defined responsibility for communications, including community outreach, collection of information on best practices, dissemination planning, and so on.
- Brief media, communications, and development offices at home institutions about projects, major milestones, and findings.
- Keep community and industry partners in the communications loop.
- Work with the Coordinating Center and NCATS on a plan for disseminating findings through the media and beyond.
- Consistently share success stories and research findings on the individual CTSA websites.
- Ensure that at least one member of the research team from each CTSA participant has had training on effective communication of scientific information.

CONCLUSIONS AND RECOMMENDATIONS

The CTSA Program has made progress in fulfilling its task of strengthening the nation's infrastructure for clinical and translational science. In implementing the CTSA Program and moving it toward CTSA 2.0, NCATS has an obligation to ensure that the significant public investment that has been made thus far is effectively contributing to the research enterprise. The IOM's 2009 report *HHS in the 21st Century* outlined a systematic approach to accountability that could be useful in leading the CTSA Program toward greater accountability and efficiency. This approach requires

- a small number of critical, measurable goals;
- clearly delineated lines of responsibility;
- quantifiable targets and time-specific milestones;
- identification of barriers and strategies to overcome them;
- a process of regular reporting and assessment;
- rewards and recognition for achieving goals;

- a clear understanding of whether progress is being made; and
- corrective action as needed (IOM, 2009).

The current clinical and translational science ecosystem presents many challenges in identifying and testing therapeutic and preventive interventions for safety and efficacy and moving them into clinical and community settings. The IOM committee believes that the CTSA Program has a major role to play in overcoming those challenges and facilitating and accelerating clinical and translational research. Meeting these tasks will necessitate a CTSA Program that meets the accountability standards outlined above, is nimble enough to be action oriented, has the ability to focus the disparate energies and talents of many institutions and individuals, and is able forge the partnerships and collaborations needed to move forward in a complex research ecosystem.

The committee urges NCATS to take a more active role in the direction of the CTSA Program and to build on its current strengths by setting clear and measurable goals, streamlining the program structure, establishing accountability and transparency, communicating its value, and instilling strong evaluation expectations.

Recommendation 1: *Strengthen NCATS Leadership of the CTSA Program*

NCATS should strengthen its leadership of the CTSA Program to advance innovative and transformative efforts in clinical and translational research. As it implements CTSA 2.0, NCATS should

- **increase active involvement in the CTSA cooperative agreements and the CTSA Consortium;**
- **conduct a strategic planning process to set measurable goals and objectives for the program that address the full spectrum of clinical and translational research;**
- **ensure that the CTSA Program as a whole actively supports the full spectrum of clinical and translational research while encouraging flexibility for each institution to build on its unique strengths;**
- **form strategic partnerships with NIH institutes and centers and with other research networks and industry;**

- establish an innovations fund through a set-aside mechanism that would be used for collaborative pilot studies and other initiatives involving CTSA institutions, other NIH institutes, and/or other public and private entities (e.g., industry, other government agencies, private foundations, community advocates and organizations);
- evaluate the program as a whole to identify gaps, weaknesses, and opportunities and create mechanisms to address them; and
- distill and widely disseminate best practices and lessons learned by the CTSA Program and work to communicate its value and accomplishments and seek opportunities for further efforts and collaborations.

Recommendation 2: *Reconfigure and Streamline the CTSA Consortium*

NCATS should reconfigure and streamline the structure of the CTSA Program by establishing a new multistakeholder NCATS-CTSA Steering Committee that would

- be chaired by a member of NCATS leadership team and have a CTSA principal investigator as vice-chair, and
- provide direction to the CTSA Coordinating Center in developing and promoting the use of available shared resources.

Recommendation 3: *Build on the Strengths of Individual CTSAs Across the Spectrum of Clinical and Translational Research*

Individual CTSAs, with the leadership of NCATS, should emphasize their particular strengths in advancing the program's broad mission and goals. In doing so, CTSAs should

- drive innovation and collaboration in methodologies, processes, tools, and resources across the spectrum of clinical and translational research;
- emphasize interdisciplinary team-based approaches in training, education, and research;

- involve patients, family members, health care providers, and other community partners in all phases of the work of the CTSA;
- strengthen collaborations across the schools and disciplines in their home institutions;
- build partnerships with industry, other research networks, community groups, and other stakeholders; and
- communicate the resources available through the CTSA Program.

Recommendation 4: *Formalize and Standardize Evaluation Processes for Individual CTSAs and the CTSA Program*

NCATS should formalize and standardize its evaluation processes for individual CTSAs and the CTSA Program. The evaluations should use clear, consistent, and innovative metrics that align with the program's mission and goals and that go beyond standard academic benchmarks of publications and number of grant awards to assess the CTSA Program and the individual CTSAs.

REFERENCES

AHRQ (Agency for Healthcare Research and Quality). 2012. *Practice-Based Research Networks.* http://pbrn.ahrq.gov (accessed March 11, 2013).

Alexander, A., J. A. Hogle, C. Kane, H. M. Parsons, and L. Phelps. 2013. *The Clinical and Translational Science Award National Evaluators Survey: Where are we now?* Submitted to the IOM Committee by D. Rubio on March 28. Available by request through the National Academies' Public Access Records Office.

Austin, C. P. 2013. *National Center for Advancing Translational Sciences: Catalyzing translational innovation.* PowerPoint presented at Meeting 3: IOM Committee to Review the CTSA Program at NCATS, Washington, DC, January 24. http://www.iom.edu/~/media/Files/Activity%20Files/Research/ http://www.iom.edu/~/media/Files/Activity%20Files/Research/CTSAReview/ 2013-JAN-24/Chris%20Austin.pdf (accessed February 13, 2013).

Briggs, J. 2012. *Evaluation of the CTSA Program.* Remarks presented at Meeting 2: IOM Committee to Review the CTSA Program at NCATS, Washington, DC, December 12.

Briggs, J., and C. P. Austin. 2012. *NCATS and the evolution of the Clinical and Translational Science Award (CTSA) Program.* PowerPoint presented at

Meeting 1: IOM Committee to Review the CTSA Program at NCATS, Washington, DC, October 29. http://www.iom.edu/~/media/Files/Activity%20Files/Research/CTSAReview/2012-OCT-29/IOM%20Briggs-Austin%20102 912.pdf (accessed February 13, 2013).

Calmbach, W. L., J. G. Ryan, L.-M. Baldwin, and L. Knox. 2012. Practice-Based Research Networks (PBRNs): Meeting the challenges of the future. *Journal of the American Board of Family Medicine* 25(5):572–576.

CTSA (Clinical and Translational Science Awards) Central. 2011a. *2011 CTSA Consortium Committee annual reports.* https://www.signup4.net/Upload/BOOZ12A/CTSA37E/File%202_2011%20CTSA%20Consortium%20Committee%20Annual%20Reports.pdf (accessed March 26, 2013).

———. 2011b. *CTSA NIAID annual summary 2011.* https://www.ctsacentral.org/sites/default/files/documents/NIAID_2011.pdf (accessed February 21, 2013).

———. 2013a. *About the CTSA Consortium.* https://www.ctsacentral.org/about-us/ctsa (accessed February 13, 2013).

———. 2013b. *Assets/Catalog.* https://www.ctsacentral.org/reports/cataloging (accessed April 2, 2013).

———. 2013c. *CKFC year in review: Communications best practices.* https://ctsacentral.org/sites/default/files/documents/%2310_Communications _year_in_review.pdf (accessed March 26, 2013).

———. 2013d. *Clinical and Translational Science Awards.* https//www.ctsacentral.org/ (accessed March 26, 2013).

———. 2013e. *Communications Key Functions Committee.* https://www.ctsa central.org/committee/communications (accessed March 26, 2013).

———. 2013f. *Evaluation Key Function Committee.* https://www.ctsacentral.org/committee/evaluation (accessed March 26, 2013).

———. 2013g. *ROCKET (Research Organization, Collaboration, and Knowledge Exchange Toolkit).* https://www.ctsacentral.org/rocket (accessed March 1, 2013).

CTSA Evaluation Key Function Committee. 2012. *Evaluation guidelines for the Clinical and Translational Science Awards (CTSAs).* Submitted to the IOM Committee by D. Rubio on March 28. Available by request through the National Academies' Public Access Records Office.

CTSA PIs (Principal Investigators). 2012. Preparedness of the CTSA's structural and scientific assets to support the mission of the National Center for Advancing Translational Sciences (NCATS). *Clinical and Translational Science* 5(2):121–129.

Curley, M. A. Q. 2013. *Future directions for using CTSA programs and resources.* PowerPoint presented at Meeting 3: IOM Committee to Review the CTSA Program at NCATS, Washington, DC, January 24. http://www.iom.edu/~/media/Files/Activity%20Files/Research/CTSAReview/2013-JAN-24/Martha%20Curley.pdf (accessed March 26, 2013).

Demichelisa, F., S. R. Setlurd, S. Banerjeee, D. Chakravartya, J. Y. H. Chend, C. X. Chena, J. Huanga, H. Beltranf, D. A. Oldridgea, N. Kitabayashia, B.

Stenzelg, G. Schaeferg, W. Horningerg, J. Bekticg, A. M. Chinnaiyanh, S. Goldenbergi, J. Siddiquih, M. M. Regank, M. Kearneyl, T. D. Soongb, D. S. Rickmana, O. Elementob, J. T. Weij, D. S. Scherri, M. A. Sandal, G. Bartschg, C. Leed, H. Klockerg, and M. A. Rubin. 2012. Identification of functionally active, low frequency copy number variants at 15q21.3 and 12q21.31 associated with prostate cancer risk. *Proceedings of the National Academy of Sciences of the United States of America* 109(17):6686–6691.

Disis, N. 2012. *CTSA strategic goal 5: Advancing T1 translational research.* PowerPoint presented at Meeting 1: IOM Committee to Review the CTSA Program at NCATS, Washington, DC, October 29. http://www.iom.edu /~/media/Files/Activity%20Files/Research/CTSAReview/2012-OCT-29/CTSA %20presentations/6-Disis%20IOM_CTSA_StrategicGoal5_Disis_10%2029 %2012.pdf (accessed March 26, 2013).

Fagnan, L. J., M. Davis, R. A. Deyo, J. J. Werner, and K. C. Stange. 2010. Linking Practice-Based Research Networks and Clinical and Translational Science Awards: New opportunities for community engagement by academic health centers. *Academic Medicine* 85(3):476–483.

Felt, U., B. Wynne, M. Callon, M. E. Goncalves, S. Jasanoff, M. Jepsen, P.-B. Joly, Z. Konopasek, S. May, C. Neubauer, A. Rip, K. Siune, A. Stirling, and M. Tallacchini. 2007. *Taking European knowledge society seriously: Report of the expert group on science and governance to the science, economy and society directorate, Directorate-General for Research, European Commission.* Luxembourg: Office for Official Publications of the European Communities. http://ec.europa.eu/research/science-society/document_library/ pdf_06/european-knowledge-society_en.pdf (accessed March 26, 2013).

Fine, J. 2012. *Translation of basic science to human studies: Advancing T1 and T2 research.* PowerPoint presented at Meeting 2: IOM Committee to Review the CTSA Program at NCATS, Washington, DC, December 12. http://www.iom.edu/~/media/Files/Activity%20Files/Research/CTSAReview /2012-DEC-12/1-4%20Jacqueline%20Fine.pdf (accessed March 26, 2013).

Frechtling, J., K. Raue, J. Michie, A. Miyaoka, and M. Spiegelman. 2012. *The CTSA national evaluation phase 1 final report.* Rockville, MD: Westat. https://www.ctsacentral.org/sites/default/files/files/CTSANationalEval_Final Report_20120416.pdf (accessed April 1, 2013).

Germino, G. G. 2012. *Opportunities for NIDDK-CTSA cooperation.* PowerPoint presented at Meeting 1: IOM Committee to Review the CTSA Program at NCATS, Washington, DC, October 29. http://www.iom.edu/~/media/Files/ Activity%20Files/Research/CTSAReview/2012-OCT-20/NIH%20presentations/ 4-%20Germino%20CTSA%20IOM%20NIDDK.pdf (accessed February 21, 2013).

Harvard College. 2012. *About eagle-i.* https://www.eagle-i.net/about (accessed March 1, 2013).

Heatwole, C., R. Bode, N. Johnson, C. Quinn, W. Martens, M. P. McDermott, N. Rothrock, C. Thornton, B. Vickrey, D. Victorson, and R. Moxley III.

2012. Patient-reported impact of symptoms in myotonic dystrophy type 1 (PRISM-1). *Neurology* 79(4):348–357.

HMO (Health Maintaince Organization) Research Network. 2013. *HMO Research Network: About our organization.* http://www.hmoresearchnetwork.org/about.htm (accessed February 28, 2013).

ICSU CFRS (International Council for Science Committee on Freedom and Responsibility in the Conduct of Science). 2010. *Advisory note: "Science communication."* http://www.icsu.org/publications/cfrs-statements/science-communication/ICSU_Sci_Commn_Adv_Note_Dec2010.pdf (accessed March 26, 2013).

IOM (Institute of Medicine). 2007. *The learning healthcare system: Workshop summary.* Washington, DC: The National Academies Press.

———. 2009. *HHS in the 21st century: Charting a new course for a healthier America.* Washington, DC: The National Academies Press.

———. 2011. *Relieving pain in America: A blueprint for transforming prevention, care, education, and research.* Washington, DC: The National Academies Press.

———. 2012. *Maximizing the impact of the Cures Acceleration Network: Workshop summary.* Washington, DC: The National Academies Press.

———. 2013a. *Responses to public input questions regarding the CTSA Program at NCATS.* Submitted to the IOM Committee between December 17, 2012–March 1, 2013. Available by request through the National Academies' Public Access Records Office.

———. 2013b. *Roundtable on Value Science-Driven Health Care.* http://www.iom.edu/Activities/Quality/VSRT.aspx (accessed April 10, 2013).

Kane, C., A. Alexander, J. A. Hogle, H. M. Parsons, and L. Phelps. 2013. *Heterogeneity at Work: Implications of the 2012 Clinical Translational Science Award Evaluators Survey: Where are we now?* Submitted to the IOM Committee by D. Rubio on March 28. Available by request through the National Academies' Public Access Records Office.

Katz, S., J. Anderson, H. Auchincloss, J. Briggs, A. Guttmacher, K. Hudson, R. Hodes, W. Koroshetz, R. Ranganathan, G. Rodgers, and S. Shurin. 2011. *NIH CTSA/NCATS Integration Working Group recommendations.* http://www.ncats.nih.gov/files/recommendations.pdf (accessed April 8, 2013).

Kaufmann, P. 2013. *NeuroNEXT.* PowerPoint presented during Conference Call Meeting 3: IOM Committee to Review the CTSA Program at NCATS, Washington, DC, January 30. http://www.iom.edu/~/media/Files/Activity%20Files/Research/CTSAReview/2013-JAN-30/Petra%20Kaufmann.pdf (accessed February 25, 2013).

Lambright, W. H. 2002. *Managing "big science": A case study of the Human Genome Project.* Arlington, VA: PriceWaterhouseCoopers Endowment for the Business of Government. http://www.businessofgovernment.org/sites/default/files/HumanGenomeProject.pdf (accessed April 18, 2013).

Lee, L. S., S. N. Pusek, W. T. McCormack, D. L. Helitzer, C. A. Martina, A. M. Dozier, J. S. Ahluwalia, L. S. Schwartz, L. M. McManus, B. D. Reynolds, E. N. Haynes, and D. M. Rubio. 2012. Clinical and translational scientist career success: Metrics for evaluation. *Clinical and Translational Science* 5(5):400–407.

McCormack, F. X., Y. Inoue, J. Moss, L. G. Singer, C. Strange, K. Nakata, A. F. Barker, J. T. Chapman, M. L. Brantly, J. M. Stocks, K. K. Brown, J. P. Lynch, III, H. J. Goldberg, L. R. Young, B. W. Kinder, G. P. Downey, E. J. Sullivan, T. V. Colby, R. T. McKay, M. M. Cohen, L. Korbee, A. M. Taveira-DaSilva, H.-S. Lee, J. P. Krischer, and B. C. Trapnell. 2011. Efficacy and safety of sirolimus in lymphangioleiomyomatosis. *New England Journal of Medicine* 364(17):1595–1606.

Michaud, M. 2012. *In muscular dystrophy, what matters to patients and doctors can differ.* http://www.urmc.rochester.edu/news/story/index.cfm?id=3567 (accessed March 1, 2013).

Miyaoka, A., M. Spiegelman, K. Raue, and J. Frechtling. 2011. *Findings from the CTSA National Evaluation Education and Training Study.* Rockville, MD: Westat. https://ctsacentral.org/sites/default/files/documents/Education TrainingReport_20111228.pdf (accessed April 1, 2013).

Mulligan, L. 2012. *Compliation of Request for Information responses from May 5, 2012.* Submitted to the IOM Committee on September 17. Available by request through the National Academies' Public Access Records Office.

NCATS (National Center for Advancing Translational Sciences). 2012a. *Clinical and Translational Science Awards factsheet.* http://www.ncats.nih. gov/files/ctsa-factsheet.pdf (accessed March 26, 2013).

———. 2012b. *FAQ about CTSA RFA-TR-12-006.* http://www.ncats.nih.gov/ research/cts/ctsa/funding/faq/faq.html (accessed March 22, 2013).

———. 2012c. *Request for information: Enhancing the Clinical and Translational Science Awards Program.* http://www.ncats.nih.gov/files/report-ctsa-rfi.pdf (accessed April 8, 2013).

———. 2013a. *About NCATS.* http://www.ncats.nih.gov/about/about.html (accessed March 26, 2013).

———. 2013b. *About the CTSA Program.* http://www.ncats.nih.gov/research/ cts/ctsa/about/about.html (accessed April 8, 2013).

———. 2013c. *NCATS: Program index.* http://www.ncats.nih.gov/about/ program-index/program-index.html (accessed March 26, 2013).

———. 2013d. *News and events: Feature stories.* http://www.ncats.nih.gov/ news-and-events/features/features.html (accessed March 26, 2013).

NCRR (National Center for Research Resources). 2009. *Progress report 2006– 2008 Clinical and Translational Science Awards: Advancing scientific discoveries nationwide to improve health.* http://www.ncats.nih.gov/files/ 2008_ctsa_progress_report.pdf (accessed March 26, 2013).

NIAID (National Institute of Allergy and Infectious Diseases). 2012. *Not-for-profit partnership with Eli Lilly and Company for TB early phase drug discovery.* http://www.niaid.nih.gov/tipics/tuberculosis/research/pages/lilly.aspx (accessed April 10, 2013).

NIH (National Institutes of Health). 2005. *RFA-RM-06-002: Institutional Clinical and Translational Science Award (U54).* http://grants.nih.gov/grants/rfa-files/RFA-RM-06-002.html (accessed February 13, 2013).

———. 2009. *RFA-RM-09-004: Institutional Clinical and Translational Science Award (U54).* http://grants.nih.gov/grants/guide/rfa-files/RFA-RM-09-004.html (accessed March 22, 2013).

———. 2011. *About NIH: Mission.* http://www.nih.gov/about/mission.htm (accessed March 26, 2013).

———. 2012a. *NIH research performance progress report (RPPR) instruction guide.* http://grants.nih.gov/grants/rppr/rppr_instruction_guide.pdf (accessed March 26, 2013).

———. 2012b. *Progress report 2009–2011 Clinical and Translational Science Awards: Foundations for accelerated discovery and efficient translation.* http://www.ncats.nih.gov/ctsa_2011 (accessed March 26, 2013).

———. 2012c. *RFA-TR-12-006: Institutional Clinical and Translational Science Award (U54).* http://grants.nih.gov/grants/guide/rfa-files/rfa-tr-12-006.html (accessed February 13, 2013).

OIG (Office of the Inspector General). 2011. *NIH administration of the Clinical and Translational Science Awards Program.* https://oig.hhs.gov/oei/reports/oei-07-09-00300.pdf (accessed April 8, 2013).

Palmer, S. E., and R. A. Schibeci. 2012. What conceptions of science communication are espoused by science research funding bodies? *Public Understanding of Science*, August 24. Published online before print, doi: 10.1177/0963662512455295.

Parsons, S. 2013. *Written comments regarding CTSA evaluations.* Submitted to the IOM Committee on February 14. Available by request through the National Academies' Public Access Records Office.

Patten, I. S., S. Rana, S. Shahul, G. C. Rowe, C. Jang, L. Liu, M. R. Hacker, J. S. Rhee, J. Mitchell, F. Mahmood, P. Hess, C. Farrell, N. Koulisis, E. V. Khankin, S. D. Burke, I. Tudorache, J. Bauersachs, F. del Monte, D. Hilfiker-Kleiner, S. A. Karumanchi, and Z. Arany. 2012. Cardiac angiogenic imbalance leads to peripartum cardiomyopathy. *Nature* 485(7398):333–338.

Patton, M. Q. 2008. *Utilization-focused evaluation.* 4th ed. Thousand Oaks, CA: SAGE Publications, Inc.

Pence, K. 2012. *Discovery of treatment for rare lung disease earns U.C. researcher a national award.* http://www.uc.edu/news/NR.aspx?id=15589 (accessed March 1, 2013).

Peterson, K. A., P. D. Lipman, C. J. Lange, R. A. Cohen, and S. Durako. 2012. Supporting better science in primary care: A description of Practice-Based Research Networks (PBRNs) in 2011. *Journal of the American Board of Family Medicine* 25(5):565–571.

Prescott, B. 2012. *Researchers uncover important clues to a dangerous complication of pregnancy.* http://www.bidmc.org/News/InResearch/2012/May/Arany_PPCM.aspx (accessed March 1, 2013).

Pulley, J. 2013. *CTSA essays and worksheets. Submitted to the NIH CTSA/NCATS Integration Working Group, July 2011.* Submitted to the IOM Committee on January 7. Available by request through the National Academies' Public Access Records Office.

Purdy, M. C. 2012. *Stroke patients benefit from carmaker's efficiency.* http://news.wustl.edu/news/Pages/24442.aspx (accessed March 1, 2013).

Raue, K., A. Miyaoka, M. Spiegelman, and J. Frechtling. 2011. *Findings from the CTSA national evaluation utilization study.* Rockville, MD: Westat. https://ctsacentral.org/sites/default/files/documents/EducationTrainingReport_20111228.pdf (accessed April 1, 2013).

Reed, J. C., E. L. White, J. Aube, C. Lindsley, M. Li, L. Sklar, and S. Schreiber. 2012. The NIH's role in accelerating translational sciences. *Nature Biotechnology* 30(1):16–19.

Reis, S. E., L. Berglund, G. R. Bernard, R. M. Califf, G. A. FitzGerald, and P. C. Johnson. 2010. Reengineering the national clinical and translational research enterprise: The strategic plan of the National Clinical and Translational Science Awards Consortium. *Academic Medicine* 85(3):463–469.

Rosenblum, D., and B. Alving. 2011. The role of the Clinical and Translational Science Awards program in improving the quality and efficiency of clinical research. *Chest* 140(3):764–767.

Rubio, D. 2013. *Evaluation Key Function Committee's outline of next steps for common metrics.* Submitted to the IOM Committee on March 28. Available by request through the National Academies' Public Access Records Office.

Rubio, D. M., D. J. del Junco, R. Bhore, C. J. Lindsell, R. A. Oster, K. M. Wittkowski, L. J.Welty, Y.-J. Lih, and D. DeMetsi. 2011a. Evaluation metrics for biostatistical and epidemiological collaborations. *Statistics in Medicine* 30(23):2767–2777.

Rubio, D. M., B. A. Primack, G. E. Switzer, C. L. Bryce, D. L. Seltzer, and W. N. Kapoor. 2011b. A comprehensive career-success model for physician-scientists. *Academic Medicine* 86(12):1571–1576.

Rubio, D. M., M. Sufian, and W. M. Trochim. 2012. Strategies for a national evaluation of the Clinical and Translational Science Awards. *Clinical and Translational Science* 5(2):138–139.

Shurin, S. B. 2012. *CTSA V. 2.0 perspective from the NLHBI.* PowerPoint presented at Meeting 1: IOM Committee to Review the CTSA Program at NCATS, Washington, DC, October 29. http://www.iom.edu/~/media/Files/Activity%20Files/Research/CTSAReview/2012-OCT-29/NIH%20presentations/2-Shurin-IOM%20CTSA%202012%2010%2018%20rev%20JW.pdf (accessed February 21, 2013).

Shuster, J. J. 2012. U.S. government mandates for clinical and translational research. *Clinical and Translational Science* 5(1):83–84.

Stanford University. 2012. *Macromolecular crystallography at SSRL: AutoDrug.* http://smb.slac.stanford.edu/research/developments/autodrug (accessed April 10, 2013).

———. 2013. *About the Stanford Synchrotron Radiation Lightsource.* http://www-ssrl.slac.stanford.edu/content/about-ssrl/about-stanford-synchrotron-radiation-lightsource (accessed April 10, 2013).

Steiner, J. F. 2013. *Written comments to IOM Committee to Review the CTSA Program at NCATS for panel presentation on January 24.* Submitted to the IOM Committee on February 21. Available by request through the National Academies' Public Access Records Office.

Steketee, M., J. Frechtling, D. Cross, and J. Schnell. 2012. *Final report on CTSA-supported publications: 2006 to 2011.* Rockville, MD: Westat.

Task Force on the Principles of Community Engagement (Clinical and Translational Science Awards Consortium Community Engagement Key Function Committee Task Force on the Principles of Community Engagement). 2011. *Principles of community engagement: Second edition.* NIH Publication No. 11-7782. http://www.atsdr.cdc.gov/community engagement/pdf/PCE_Report_508_FINAL.pdf (accessed April 2, 2013).

Tsai, Y., S. E. McPhillips, T. M. McPhillips, A. González, and S. M. Soltis. 2012. *AutoDrug: An automated pipeline for drug discovery at the Stanford Synchrotron Radiation Lightsource (SSRL).* http://smb.slac.stanford.edu/research/developments/autodrug/handout.html (accessed April 10, 2013).

University of Rochester. 2012. *CTSA IP: Intellectual Property information exchange.* http://www.ctsaip.org (accessed March 1, 2013).

Vanderbilt University. 2011. *Vanderbilt University Medical Center awarded $20 million to coordinate science consortium.* http://www.mc.vanderbilt.edu/news/releases.php?release=2152 (accessed April 10, 2013).

———. 2012. *ResearchMatch.* https://www.researchmatch.org (accessed March 1, 2013).

———. 2013a. *IRBshare.* https://www.irbshare.org (accessed February 13, 2013).

———. 2013b. *REDCap (Research Electronic Data Capture).* http://project-redcap.org (accessed March 1, 2013).

VIVO. 2013. *About VIVO.* http://vivoweb.org/about (accessed March 1, 2013).

Volkow, N. 2012. *Building drug abuse research at NIDA in cooperation with the CTSA consortium.* PowerPoint presented during Conference Call Meeting 1: IOM Committee to review the CTSA program at NCATS, Washington, DC, November 19. http://www.iom.edu/~/media/Files/Activity%20Files/Research/CTSAReview/2012-NOV-19/Nora%20Volkow.pdf (accessed February 22, 2013).

Wadman, M. 2010. NIH encourages translational collaboration with industry. *Nature Reviews Drug Discovery* 9(4):255–256.

Weiss, L. 2012. *Written comments to IOM Committee to Review the CTSA Program at NCATS for panel presentation.* Submitted to the IOM Committee on October 29. Available by request through the National Academies' Public Access Records Office.

Westat. 2011. *Report on field visits to CTSAs.* Rockville, MD: Westat. https://www.ctsacentral.org/sites/default/files/documents/FieldVisit_Final Report_2011June.pdf (accessed April 1, 2013).

Woods, L. 2012. *Two genetic deletions in human genome linked to the development of aggressive prostate cancer.* http://weill.cornell.edu/news/releases/wcmc/wcmc_2012/04_09_12.shtml (accessed March 1, 2013).

Zerhouni, E. A. 2005. Translational and clinical science—time for a new vision. *New England Journal of Medicine* 353(15):1621–1623.

4

Crosscutting Topics

The Clinical and Translational Science Awards (CTSA) Program has demonstrated progress in three crosscutting domains that the Institute of Medicine (IOM) committee believes are integral to effectively advancing clinical and translational science: training and education, community engagement, and child health research. These efforts, along with the program's contributions in building infrastructure and providing a range of research resources, make the CTSA Program a unique national resource within the clinical and translational research landscape. As with all such activities, each of these functions can be strengthened in a variety of ways. The committee provides a brief overview of each of these areas, followed by its recommendations for next steps.

TRAINING AND EDUCATION

The health needs of the nation call for a generation of scientists trained in "interdisciplinary, transformative translational research" (Meyers et al., 2012, p. 132; Van Hartesveldt et al., 2008) and in the leadership and team skills to engage in effective collaborative partnerships. A major challenge in rapidly translating research findings into health care practice is the concomitant need for support of clinician scientists in order to overcome the growing divide between clinical (M.D.) and research (Ph.D.) careers (Roberts et al., 2012). Further, emerging and growing areas of research (including comparative-effectiveness and community-engaged research) are emphasizing skills and collaborations integral to both clinical and translational research.

Background and Context

Sustaining a vibrant clinical and translational research enterprise in the future depends on building and retaining a diverse research workforce. Education and training in clinical and translational research are priorities for the CTSA Program. All CTSA institutions are expected to provide robust postgraduate training (NIH, 2012c), and many have extensive training programs that often include undergraduate and predoctoral student training as well as training for research staff and community collaborators. In addition, the CTSA Consortium has identified "training and career development of clinical and translational scientists" as a consortium strategic goal and has devoted considerable resources to enhancing the effectiveness of training and education programs across institutions (CTSA Central, 2013a,e).

CTSA Training Awards and Programs

Since the inception of the CTSA Program, the training of new clinical and translational science investigators has been an integral part of the program. The KL2 Mentored Clinical Research Scholar Program is a required part of all individual CTSAs (NIH, 2012c). This career development program provides awardees who have a doctoral degree (M.D., Ph.D., or equivalent) with formal research training experience and funding support to help them become independent investigators (NCATS, 2013). The TL1 Clinical Research Training Program provides an introduction to clinical and translational research to pre- and postdoctoral candidates or others who want to learn more about these types of research. For example, the TL1 program can provide medical students with a structured year-long research opportunity. In fiscal year (FY) 2011, 501 scholars participated in the KL2 program, and 469 trainees participated in the TL1 program through the CTSA Program (Collier, 2013a). Many CTSAs offer a master's level degree in clinical and translational research.

In 2011, Westat provided its findings from an online survey of CTSA-supported scholars, trainees, and mentors from CTSAs funded between 2006 and 2010 (Miyaoka et al., 2011). A total of 665 mentors (56 percent response rate) and 553 scholars and trainees (43 percent response rate) completed the surveys. Overall, the results were positive. Mentors reported providing a range of support in key areas for career development, and they reported benefits to their own professional development. Scholars and trainees reported developing more skills and having enhanced opportunities for career development. Areas for improvement included the need for greater diversity among mentors, scholars, and trainees; increased emphasis on team science; and additional focus on the development of skills related to technology transfer, commercialization, and communicating with policy makers. Box 4-1 presents a few highlights from this evaluation.

CTSA Consortium Efforts on Training and Education

At the consortium level, the Strategic Goal Committee on Training and Career Development has developed and disseminated core competencies in clinical and translational science for master's degree students (CTSA Central, 2011), as well as core competencies in specific areas, including child health translational research, T1 research, academia-industry drug development, and medical device innovation and technology transfer (CTSA Central, 2011).

BOX 4-1
Selected Highlights from the CTSA National Evaluation
Education and Training Study

- CTSAs are engaging scholars and trainees across the spectrum of translational research (21 percent basic biomedical research; 52 percent clinical research; 26 percent postclinical research).
- Trainees report positive experiences in educational activities. For example, 92 percent responded that building relationships with mentors was useful; 96 percent were positive about working as a member of a research team.
- Evidence of success was found in obtaining R01 funding (47 percent of R01 applications were funded). The rate of submission was low, however (16 percent of scholars or trainees reported submitting an R01 application).
- Clear benefits were noted by mentors (97 percent of mentors rated their experience as positive) and trainees or scholars (83 percent assessed their levels of training and expertise in clinical research as moderate or high after participating in the CTSA Program, compared with a baseline 33 percent).
- Most scholars and trainees reported serving as the PI on their first (79 percent) and second (72 percent) grant/award applications.

SOURCE: Miyaoka et al., 2011.

The additional goals of the strategic goal committee are to provide CTSA-wide access to training resources, develop a core curriculum, implement a mentoring training program that shares best practices, and develop metrics and criteria for recognizing success and achieving career promotion in clinical and translational research (CTSA Central, 2013e).

Opportunities and Next Steps

CTSA 2.0 should build on the successes of the training and education components of individual CTSAs and the consortium-level work. This calls for new and innovative training and education approaches and methodologies. Training and education efforts are a prime area for collaboration with NIH institutes and centers to monitor, track, and adopt best practices and successful models in education, mentoring, and career development.

Presentations to the IOM committee and peer-reviewed publications highlighted a range of innovative training opportunities that could be brought to scale for greater impact. These include training and education across the educational spectrum (i.e., from undergraduate to postgraduate levels) and learning opportunities for community partners, faculty, and research administrators. Academic training options also exist across levels of intensity, from individual courses to certificate programs to advanced degrees.

Innovative Curricula and Team-Based Education and Training

The excitement and the challenge of clinical and translational science is that it requires approaches to training and education that are outside of traditional scientific fields. The focus on a truly team-based and interdisciplinary approach to science requires collaborations that go far beyond lip service and necessitates relationship building between and among professional schools (e.g., medicine, nursing, business, law, engineering, public health), as well as with a range of community partners (from patients and families to health care providers). Learning in this field is often through and by experience. Further, the topics to be covered stretch beyond traditional ones to include, for example, entrepreneurship, intellectual property, regulatory science, health equity, unconscious bias, and community engagement.

In a number of CTSAs, innovative efforts to develop new courses and curricula are already under way. For example, the CTSA partnership in which the University of Washington is involved implements a team-based translational educational program with a clinical and translational research boot camp workshop and several active seminar series, including a monthly clinical research education series focused on conveying practical information and tools (ITHS, 2013). The goal is for translational scientists to have competencies related to key questions at each phase of the translational research cycle, including

- Which problems will we tackle? (discovery phase);
- How will the handoff happen to move discoveries into human studies? (development phase);
- Can we scale up into clinics or communities? (delivery phase); and
- How will we know we are making a real impact? (outcomes phase) (Edwards, 2013; Kelley et al., 2012).

In another innovative training model, the University of Pennsylvania offers a variety of training options for undergraduates; predoctoral, graduate, and postdoctoral students; fellows; clinical residents; and faculty with several types of certificates or advanced degrees offered. In addition to general training in clinical and translational science, this program offers a concentration in translational therapeutics that includes public-private partnerships for industry internships and training in intellectual property and commercialization (Meagher, 2011; University of Pennsylvania ITMAT, 2013).

CTSA 2.0 should build on these and other innovative training and education programs that are bridging the gap between the basic and clinical sciences. Emphasis on experiential and team-based learning and incorporating topics outside the traditional realm will provide the solid foundation needed to spur clinical and translational research. CTSAs have the potential both to create learning cultures that embrace innovative teaching methods and content (e.g., gaming, flipped classrooms,[1] mini-institutes) and to disseminate those innovations rapidly and effectively.

---

[1]Flipped classrooms typically offer instruction online and doing homework in the classroom.

Effective Mentoring and Coaching

An emphasis on effective mentoring has also been a strength and integral component of CTSA training programs. In 2008, the CTSA Education and Career Development Key Function Committee established a Mentor Working Group that has identified several key elements of successful mentoring programs: mentor selection and support, alignment of mentor and mentee expectations, mentor training, evaluation, and feedback (Fleming et al., 2012).

Recent surveys and interviews found that the active mentoring programs that are in place at CTSAs for the KL2 awards differ widely regarding policies on selecting mentors, criteria to qualify as a mentor, and processes to evaluate the mentoring relationships (Huskins et al., 2011; Silet et al., 2010; Tillman et al., 2013). Programs also varied on the formality of the mentoring program, with 30 percent reporting the use of mentoring contracts (Huskins et al., 2011). Two-thirds of the mentoring programs reported requiring or encouraging mentees to have multidisciplinary mentors, with mentors or the program taking the lead to coordinate this effort to varying degrees (Silet et al., 2010). The same survey found that CTSA institutions infrequently provide tangible support for mentors, such as salary support, institutional recognition, and research support.

Successful mentoring practices should be disseminated across the CTSA Program. While avoiding the pitfalls of just checking boxes, the CSTA Program should consider developing metrics for how mentoring is evaluated. Mentoring is not an inherent skill for many people, but it can be developed by training and alignment of incentives. Positive mentoring experiences appear to be linked to strong relationships with individual mentors. The time commitment made to mentoring should be recognized in decisions on the mentor's career advancement.

A new initiative being announced by the NIH Common Fund and the National Research Mentoring Network offers opportunities for focused efforts on mentoring and will aim to provide mentoring standards, training for mentors, and opportunities to increase the diversity of participants involved in being a mentor or mentee (NIH, 2013b). CTSA Program participation in this network could be a benefit to furthering CTSA mentoring opportunities. Consideration could be given to trans-CTSA mentorships where predoctoral students in one institution would have mentors in multiple CTSA institutions, thereby sharing specific expertise, creating venues for innovative partnerships, and opening up a potential pipeline for recruitment across institutions when their predoctoral training is completed.

Flexibility and Focus

Consistency in key components of training and education, such as core competencies and standards, can be balanced with flexibility in the elements and focus of the training experiences. Input received by the IOM committee from those who had participated in the CTSA training programs identified many positive aspects of the training experience, including protected time to develop a programmatic research agenda and grant proposals; exposure to multidisciplinary perspectives; committed mentoring relationships; high-quality courses, seminars, and workshops; support for participation in national conferences; and access to pilot grant funding and core resources (Ceglia, 2013; IOM, 2013; Shackelford, 2013). Areas of concern included the lack of awareness of the range of core resources available through the CTSA and the extensive time commitment for completing an advanced degree in the CTSA institutions that require this as part of the training program.[2]

In moving to CTSA 2.0, the IOM committee urges increased flexibility in training and education programs. The extensive list of competencies identified by the strategic goal committee (CTSA Central, 2011) offers many potential areas for program development. The objective should be to personalize training experiences to meet the needs and goals of individuals and focus on competency rather than on the absolute requirement of obtaining a master's or other advanced degree. This flexibility will be valuable in attracting and retaining KL2 scholars and TL1 trainees and may be particularly pertinent to clinician-scientists, who can play a major role in the clinical and translational research enterprise.

Disseminating Education and Training Materials

The transformation of training and education is possible only through the dissemination of successful approaches and practices. Several efforts are under way to provide online repositories of CTSA training and education modules and materials. The Virtual University through the Uni-

---

[2]CTSA institutions have the flexibility to decide how to structure their career development programs. In some CTSAs the KL2 participants are required to obtain a master's degree as part of the KL2 program, and the degree is optional at other CTSA sites (Collier, 2013b).

versity of Iowa offers access to online courses relevant to clinical and translational sciences (University of Iowa ICTS, 2013). The National CTSA Educational Resource Program, developed by the University of Rochester's Clinical and Translational Science Institute, provides links to educational modules from a number of CTSAs (University of Rochester CTSI, 2013). Online access to course materials on mentoring is available through the Mentor Development Program at the University of California, San Francisco (University of California San Francisco CTSI, 2013).

Notable in the information obtained by the IOM committee regarding training and education is frequent sharing of courses, seminars, workshops, and other resources among the CTSA sites and other training and education programs within institutions. This sharing enhances cross-disciplinary training within individual institutions and across the CTSA institutions. The IOM committee notes that similarities in core curricula highlight opportunities for improving efficiencies in training as well as for exposing scholars and trainees to expertise in areas of particular strength from one CTSA institution to another.

Increasing Diversity and Growth of the Clinical and Translational Research Workforce

To date, scholars, trainees, and mentors in CTSA programs lack diversity. The Westat evaluation showed that most mentors are white males, and most scholars and trainees are white females (Miyaoka et al., 2011). Bringing the brightest minds to research, which is critical for new discoveries to improve health, depends on creating a training and education environment that attracts and retains a diverse pool of scientists. Innovative education programs such as Harvard University's Summer Clinical and Translational Research Program for undergraduate scholars have the potential to create a pipeline of diverse clinical and translational scientists (Harvard Medical School DCP, 2013), particularly if partnerships are formed with colleges and universities that traditionally serve racial and ethnic minority students.

Opportunities may also be available for CTSAs to connect with STEM (science, technology, engineering, and mathematics) initiatives within and across institutions. CTSAs need to take full advantage of efforts sponsored by the NIH and others to build diversity, and, moreover, they should lead in the implementation of these initiatives. An example is the BUILD Program (Building Infrastructure Leading to Diversity) and the National Research Mentoring Network (NIH, 2013a). The National

Institute on Minority Health and Health Disparities sponsors Research Centers in Minority Institutions (RCMI), which provide additional opportunities for ongoing collaborations with the CTSA Program, particularly with the RCMI Translational Research Network (NIMHD, 2013).

Metrics and Incentives for Careers in Clinical and Translational Research

Traditional metrics have been used for the most part to measure the success of CTSA training and education programs. These metrics include

- number of scholars and trainees;
- conversion rate from K (training) to R (independent investigator) grants;
- number of publications; and
- number and types of degrees completed (Miyaoka et al., 2011).

These metrics do not measure or provide incentives for the team-based and interdisciplinary approaches needed to accomplish clinical and translational research. If the CTSAs are to be centers for innovations in clinical and translational research, they should also lead in innovations in mentoring and its evaluation, including assessment of the professional career trajectory of those who have participated in the training programs, creation of networking opportunities, active participation in national professional organizations, and commitment or intention of the scholars and trainees to engage in clinical and translational research.

Two groups within the CTSA Program have begun related efforts to examine the components of career success for clinical and translation scientists and the metrics needed to assess individual and organizational progress. The Research on Careers Workgroup at the University of Pittsburgh identified personal factors (e.g., demographic and psychosocial factors, research experience) and organizational factors (e.g., training opportunities, financial resources, balance of research and clinical responsibilities) contributing to career success for physician-scientists (Rubio et al., 2011). This information can provide training programs with insights on critical areas for working with scholars, trainees, and mentors. The CTSA Education Evaluation Working Group identified validated metrics and measures for assessing personal and organizational determinants of career success for clinical and translational scientists (Lee et al., 2012).

NCATS and individual CTSAs have the opportunity to lead changes in how training and education programs are assessed and in instituting incentives for the recognition and promotion of those involved. The traditional benchmarks for academic promotion and advancement are focused on individuals and products (e.g., publications, new grants). New benchmarks that value team-based efforts and collaborative approaches are needed to complement these traditional metrics. Changing those measures will be challenging because it is difficult to assess the depth or substance of collaborations. Identifying the right measures and incentives is a major challenge for CTSA 2.0. Examples of relevant measures might include the following:

- evidence of interdisciplinary collaborations and of teams that cross disciplines and include community partners;
- increases in the number of training and educational opportunities outside of KL2 and TL1;
- increases in the number and level of involvement of community-based health care providers and other community stakeholders in the CTSA's activities;
- higher satisfaction with mentoring relationships and increases in trained mentors; and
- the extent of public communication and knowledge transfer.

Expanding Training Opportunities

To date, CTSAs have made substantial progress in developing graduate and postdoctoral training in clinical and translational research. In addition to sustaining and building on those efforts, further work is needed to expand those opportunities, including training and continuing education for faculty, professional staff, and community partners. For example, substantive involvement of community partners in clinical and translational science provides the opportunity for education in research methodologies and design, policy and regulatory aspects of clinical trials, and dissemination of clinical innovations.

Community partner training generally appears rather informal across CTSA institutions. One example of a formal program is the Community Engaged Scholars Program developed and implemented by the South Carolina Clinical and Translational Research Center for Community Health Partnerships. This 18-month program focuses on developing competencies in community-based participatory research among teams that must include at least one academic and one community partner. Program components include monthly sessions focused on problem-based learning, mentorship, and funding for pilot projects. An early evaluation found the program successfully recruited and retained teams that identified and implemented community-based translational research pilot studies (Andrews et al., 2012).

As CTSAs continue to develop as strong networks of diverse stakeholders, there will be important opportunities to provide all participants with training and education on clinical and translational science. Meaningful involvement and collaboration among diverse groups require some common starting points, and CTSAs are the prime location for the training needed.

Conclusions and Recommendation

Training and education in clinical and translational research is a core element of all CTSAs. To date, significant progress has been made in identifying core competencies and in developing curricula in clinical and translational research. CTSA 2.0 will require further efforts to develop and implement innovative education and training approaches that emphasize the unique aspects of clinical and translational science. The full range of stakeholders needs to have expertise so they can contribute fully to the accelerated development and implementation of new therapies, preventive measures, and devices to improve health.

Recommendation 5: *Advance Innovation in Education and Training Programs*

The CTSA Program should provide training, mentoring, and education as essential core elements. To better prepare the next generation of a diverse clinical and translational science workforce, the CTSA Program should

- **emphasize innovative education and training models and methodologies, which include a focus on team science, leadership, community engagement, and entrepreneurship;**
- **disseminate high-quality online offerings for essential core courses for use in CTSA and other institutions;**

- champion the reshaping of career development pathways for researchers involved in the conduct of clinical and translational science; and
- ensure flexible and personalized training experiences that offer optional advanced degrees.

COMMUNITY ENGAGEMENT

Effective translational research requires effective community engagement across the full spectrum of research from basic science and first-in-human studies (T0–T1) to community and population health research (T4). For the purposes of this report, the IOM committee has adopted a widely cited CDC definition of community engagement: "the process of working collaboratively with and through groups of people affiliated by geographic proximity, special interest, or similar situations to address issues affecting the well-being of those people" (CDC and ATSDR, 1997). The committee considers that the term "community" can include all stakeholders connected to clinical and translational research. This broad definition encompasses the people who are served by the individual CTSAs, including patients and families, community organizations, and disease advocates, as well as clinicians and health professionals, including physicians, nurses, dentists, nutritionists, social workers, and many others. The committee also recognizes the "research community," which includes the full range of researchers—basic, clinical, and locally based researchers who work both inside and outside of academic settings. In this section of the chapter, however, when the word "community" is used, it denotes the people who seek and provide health care in community, academic, and private settings, as well as individuals and organizations working in communities to improve the health and well-being of local populations.

Community engagement in clinical and translational research varies in terms of both level of engagement and the stage(s) of research in which public participants are involved. The type of research in which community members are most deeply involved is community-based participatory research (CBPR), which engages local participants as partners and involves them in shared leadership roles throughout the entire research process, from concept development to protocol design to dissemination of the research findings. The least involvement includes outreach mechanisms that are primarily unidirectional and may entail a researcher providing information about research results or ongoing research in the region (Hood et al., 2010; Task Force on the Principles of Community Engagement, 2011).

Communities can contribute to the full range of clinical and translational research in important ways that are not always recognized (see Box 4-2). For example, partnerships with community representatives can identify community health needs and priorities, provide critical input and data on clinically relevant questions, develop culturally appropriate clinical research protocols, promote successful enrollment and retention of research participants, and, ultimately, disseminate and implement research results more effectively. In addition, community engagement at early stages of research helps to ensure that ethical considerations are taken into account and facilitates early establishment of trust (Horowitz et al., 2009; Martinez et al., 2012; Woolf, 2008).

The benefits of community engagement therefore are numerous and can lead to a more robust research enterprise, stronger community support for research and research funding, and attract more, and more diverse, young people to careers in research (Freeman and Seifer, 2013; Staley, 2009; Task Force on the Principles of Community Engagement, 2011; Yarborough et al., 2012).

BOX 4-2
Examples of Community Engagement in Clinical and Translational Research

For basic research (T0–T1), communities and patient advocacy organizations can play a vital role in identifying research areas, providing resources and specimens to support research, and putting a human face on the diseases and disorders being studied. For example, the Hermansky-Pudlak Syndrome (HPS) Network is a nonprofit advocacy organization that supports patients and families with HPS, a genetic disorder associated with albinism, bleeding, visual impairment, inflammatory bowel disease, and pulmonary fibrosis (HPS Network, 2013). The HPS Network has worked to identify research questions, recruit researchers, build partnerships, and fund research studies that have used animal models to investigate cell lines in the lungs of mice with HPS that are most susceptible to pulmonary fibrosis (Young et al., 2007). Likewise, PXE International, Inc., a nonprofit advocacy organization, provides support for research and for individuals and families affected by pseudoxanthoma elasticum (PXE), a genetic disorder that can lead to changes in vision, skin elasticity, and the cardiovascular and gastrointestinal systems. To expand research in this area, PXE International worked with patients and families to establish a biobank of blood and tissue samples made available to researchers conducting genetic research (PXE International,

2012). Both of these organizations work to bridge the gap between patients and basic science researchers studying these rare disorders.

In the clinical trial phases of clinical and translational research (T2–T3), community organizations can play a significant role in developing appropriate research protocols, helping researchers understand the needs and culture of the patient population, and recruiting prospective research participants. The HIV/AIDS community has played an active role in research since the beginning of the HIV/AIDS epidemic. To facilitate these interactions, the National Institute of Allergy and Infectious Diseases (NIAID) made Community Advisory Boards (CABs) a requirement for all HIV/AIDS clinical trial networks and sites it funds (Community Partners, 2009). The CABs have provided a venue for dialog between the community and clinical researchers and provided an opportunity for community representatives to participate in trial design and recruitment. NIAID continues to make community engagement a priority in HIV/AIDS research by supporting a number of other mechanisms to foster community participation in clinical trials. For example, the Legacy Project and Community Partners work to build trust, cultivate partnerships, and ensure effective community representation in clinical trials with an emphasis on engaging underrepresented communities (Dieffenbach, 2011; HANC, 2013a,b; Kagan et al., 2012).

Community engagement is an inherent part of community health and population health research (T4). The Healing Canoe Project is an example of a multiphase collaborative project that applies the community-based participatory research model. The project is a partnership between the Suquamish Tribe, the Port Gamble S'Klallam Tribe, and the Alcohol and Drug Abuse Institute (ADAI) at the University of Washington and is funded by the National Center on Minority Health and Health Disparities (Healing of the Canoe, 2013; Thomas et al., 2010). The first phase of the project (2005–2008) focused on the partnership between ADAI and the Suquamish Tribe. During that phase, researchers conducted a community assessment that involved interviews and focus groups to identify needs related to substance abuse prevention and cultural identity among youth. They used a team-based approach to develop a curriculum that blended elder community members' experiences, the community's traditions and culture, cognitive-behavioral skills, and information about alcohol and drugs. The second phase of the project (2008–2013) is continuing this work and using the same methods to adapt the project for the Port Gamble S'Klallam Tribe (Healing of the Canoe, 2013; Thomas et al., 2010).

An array of information has been developed on the principles, best practices, and need and potential for community engagement in all aspects of the research process, and studies have delineated the best methods to achieve authentic engagement, including defining community, identifying partners, learning the etiquette of community engagement, building sustainable networks of community engagement researchers, developing new engagements, and refining translation and dissemination plans (Hatcher and Nicola, 2008; IOM, 2012a; Michener et al., 2012).

Nevertheless, as noted by Hood and colleagues (2010), "to date, there is a paucity of research about the prevalence of community engagement in research, especially among clinical and translational research studies traditionally funded by NIH" (p. 19). This report will not review the literature on best practices and principles of community engagement. The committee recognizes the many valuable contributions to the field made by such reports as *Principles of Community Engagement* (Task Force on the Principles of Community Engagement, 2011), *Communities as Partners in Cancer Clinical Trials: Changing Research, Practice and Policy* (ENACCT and CCPH, 2008), and *Recommendations for Community Involvement in National Institute of Allergy and Infectious Diseases HIV/AIDS Clinical Trials Research* (Community Partners, 2009), along with the work conducted, for example, through the CTSA Program, the Community-Campus Partnerships for Health (CCPH), the Centers for Disease Control and Prevention, the Patient-Centered Outcomes Research Institute, and various NIH institutes and centers.

The CTSA Program and Community Engagement

Community engagement was identified as a priority area from the earliest stages of the CTSA Program and became a required key function for CTSA sites as administered by the National Center for Research Resources (NIH, 2009a,b, 2012b). Shifts in the requirements of the most recent RFA, which were made to provide increased flexibility for the individual CTSAs, have caused concern among some community organizations and advocacy groups that community engagement is being downplayed (CCPH, 2012b; Seifer, 2013; Thomas, 2013). Although the key functions that were previously required are no longer explicit requirements, the recent RFA does indicate that all CTSAs must have core resources across the full spectrum of translational research. It also encourages individual CTSAs to build a program to "meet the needs of their own investigative and public communities and to develop and build upon unique institutional and community strengths," which implies some level of necessary community engagement (NIH, 2012c).

The CTSA Consortium has adopted a set of competencies for clinical and translational research that includes community engagement as a core competency (CTSA Central, 2011). The "Frequently Asked Questions" section of the recent RFA refers to future solicitations in 2014 and highlights community engagement as an area of interest for NCATS

(NCATS, 2012a). NCATS staff confirmed that "the NCATS Advisory Council approved concept clearance for [a new initiative titled] 'Strengthening Community-Engaged Research in the CTSA Program' at its September 2012 meeting" but indicated that "no decision has been made on what form this initiative will take" (Parsons, 2013). Initial information regarding future partnerships with NIH institutes and centers for demonstration projects also highlights community engagement as an area of focus (NCATS, 2012a).

On October 15, 2012, NCATS released an RFI focused on how community engagement research could be enhanced through the CTSA Program with the end goal being "the development of a research agenda that would leverage the community engagement capability of the CTSA institutions to solve critical roadblocks in the translational research process" and that would build "on the CTSA community engagement projects, collaborations, and infrastructure to facilitate the conduct of translational research" (NIH, 2012b). The RFI asked for stakeholder input on possible research questions and opportunities to advance research, tools, and techniques for community engagement and on the role of community engagement and community-based participatory research in clinical and translational research. The responses to the RFI were still being reviewed by NCATS just prior to the IOM committee's final meeting in March 2013, but the authors of a few of the responses shared their comments with the committee and emphasized a commitment to community engagement and a continued need for it within the CTSA Program (CCPH, 2012a; Emmons, 2012; Parsons, 2013).

The initial commitment to community engagement within the CTSA Program should be commended. However, NCATS's vision for how community engagement will be a part of the CTSA Program moving forward remains unclear. Although indications point to community engagement remaining an important feature of the program, there are serious concerns that if it is not an explicit requirement for all CTSAs, it may fade in importance. These concerns were expressed clearly by the CCPH in its response to the RFI on community engagement, highlighted at the IOM committee's January 2013 meeting. The CCPH sees "troubling signs that CTSAs are already responding to a perceived lack of NCATS support for community engagement" by reducing resources supporting community engagement and putting a hold on community engagement activities (CCPH, 2012a). In developing its plans for implementing the CTSA Program and how community engagement will fit within it, NCATS must carefully consider unintended consequences of its decisions in terms of developing and sustaining fragile partnerships that have been and continue to be built.

Progress in Community Engagement

Because community engagement has been a required part of the CTSA Program, individual CTSAs and the CTSA Consortium have dedicated time and resources to building partnerships with community organizations and representatives, developing and sharing tools and resources to facilitate community engagement, educating researchers and communities, building trust, and engaging communities in the research process. The CTSA Consortium has two main committees focused on community engagement—Strategic Goal Committee 4, which focuses on "enhancing the health of our communities and the nation," and the Community Engagement Key Function Committee, which has eight working groups devoted to a range of related areas, including practice-based research network collaborations, health policy, resource development, and community partner integration (CTSA Central, 2013c). These two committees work "to identify and develop effective partnerships among researchers and community stakeholders" and "to implement a successful broad plan of community and practice engagement among the CTSA sites by sharing knowledge, expertise and resources" (CTSA Central, 2013c,f). These committees and working groups have facilitated the development of a range of tools and resources for CTSAs and researchers that promote effective community engagement (see Box 4-3) (Brady, 2012).

In addition to activities facilitated through the CTSA Consortium, individual CTSAs are making progress in community engagement efforts. A recent survey of involvement of community representatives in CTSA activities found that, of the 47 CTSAs responding (out of 60 surveyed), almost 90 percent have established a community advisory board (Spofford et al., 2012). However, these boards are used primarily to advise the community engagement cores at the CTSAs and are involved to a lesser extent in advising CTSA leadership. The survey also revealed few opportunities for community representatives to participate in leadership roles beyond those within the community engagement core or on CTSA leadership committees.

To fully engage community representatives throughout the CTSA Program, strategies should be developed and implemented that integrate community representatives beyond community engagement projects. This effort should include having community representatives actively participate in leadership and governance committees of the CTSA Program and individual CTSAs and obtaining substantive input from them on how to improve community engagement.

BOX 4-3
Examples of Community Engagement Tools

- *Sentinel Network for Community-Based Participatory Research:* a collaborative project with five CTSAs and several partner organizations that works to identify strategies to increase community participation in clinical research through education and referrals. Since the start of the program, more than 5,000 individuals have been surveyed on topics related to barriers to participating in research, local health concerns and needs, and the types of research in which they would be willing to participate (NIH, 2012a).

- *Community Engagement Consultative Service (CECS):* a two-phase program that provides consultations and referrals to help individual CTSAs and researchers "develop the knowledge, skills, and attitudes to successfully engage with internal and external groups and communities" (Carter-Edwards et al., 2013, p. 34). Phase I of the program tested the feasibility and utilization of the service, and Phase II paired individual CTSAs with consultants to promote improvements in community engagement (Carter-Edwards et al., 2013; Duke Center for Community Research, 2013).

- *Community Research Utilities and Support (CORUS):* an online database designed for sharing resources and tools related to community-engaged research. Resources include evaluation tools and strategies, education modules, stakeholder registries, communications tools, and ethics resources (Indiana University CTSI, 2012).

- *The Research Toolkit (formerly known as PRIMER or Partnership-driven Resources to IMprove and Enhance Research):* an online library of available resources and tools meant to facilitate multisite research involving community organizations and PBRNs. The toolkit is organized by phase of research to provide investigators with a complete guide. A collaborative team of researchers that included members from three CTSAs, PBRNs, and the HMO Research Network developed the toolkit (Dolor et al., 2011; Research Toolkit, 2012).

- *Principles of Community Engagement:* an almost 200-page primer developed by a task force of the Community Engagement Key Function Committee. This resource compiles definitions, principles, examples, and best practices, along with challenges and mechanisms for evaluating community engagement (Task Force on the Principles of Community Engagement, 2011).

As noted by the NIH CTSA/NCATS Integration Working Group, "The CTSA requirement for community outreach has led many institutions to develop or strengthen community-based research, though this is one of the most highly variable aspects of the CTSAs" (Katz et al., 2011). Examples of community engagement efforts at individual CTSAs are provided in Box 4-4.

BOX 4-4
Examples of Community Engagement Projects at CTSAs

- *Chicago Consortium for Community Engagement:* a partnership between Northwestern University, the University of Chicago, and the University of Illinois at Chicago designed to facilitate coordination and synergy in order to enhance the capacity of each of the institutions for community engagement through a range of activities, including having regular meetings for the Chicago community-based participatory research network, providing education and training for researchers and community organizations, developing a map of research opportunities across the city, and hosting a citywide summit to discuss challenges and opportunities for improving the health of Chicagoans (C3, 2013; CTSA Central, 2013b).

- *Clinical and Translational Science Collaborative of Cleveland at Case Western Reserve University:* a collaboration of support of local PBRNs with stabilizing funding and micropilot grants that have supported more than 115 projects. One PBRN encompasses 50 practices and is supported by the Robert Wood Johnson Foundation. In 3 years the work of this PBRN has lowered hemoglobin A1c levels by 1 percentage point—enough to reduce risks of complications—in a population of 27,000 patients with type II diabetes (Case Western Reserve University CTSC, 2012; Pulley, 2013a).

- *University of Cincinnati's Community Leaders Institute:* a 6-week training program for community leaders designed to "assist agencies that engage and empower communities to reduce health, social and educational disparities in leveraging funding and learning how to use data to improve services and programs." Since the program started in 2010, 41 community leaders have completed it. The first cohort of the program, which had 9 people, has secured more than $1.3 million in grants for their community organizations. Previous participants included individuals from such diverse local organizations as the YMCA of Greater Cincinnati, the Cincinnati Health Department, Lincoln Heights Missionary Baptist Church, and Sickle Cell Affected Families of Greater Cincinnati (Pulley, 2013a; University of Cincinnati CCTST, 2013).

- *Scripps Translational Science Institute Community Engagement Program:* a partnership with the Scripps Whittier Diabetes Institute developed to improve prevention and treatment strategies for diabetes in a high-risk population—individuals in the San Diego area with Mexican

ancestry. To achieve these goals, the program leverages genomic sciences, wireless technologies, established community partnerships, and
culturally appropriate approaches to community education and health
care. The program also includes a diabetes gene bank and a study on
gestational diabetes (NIH, 2012a; STSI, 2013).

Although many compelling examples of community engagement exist, assessing how widespread community engagement really is and at what level it is occurring is difficult. Hood and colleagues (2010) conducted a survey to establish a baseline of community engagement across research being funded by the NIH at one midwestern university with a CTSA. Of the 194 NIH-funded studies (out of 480) for which responses were received, fewer than half (43 percent) included community engagement activities at any level. Of the studies that included a community engagement component, only 17 percent reported meaningful community engagement that involved significant collaborative actions. These results prompted the investigators to recommend that CTSAs clarify the goals of community engagement and determine "whether community engagement programs should strive to increase the number of authentic CBPR studies, increase less intensive community engagement activities in all NIH-funded research, or both" (Hood et al., 2010, p. 22).

Metrics and Evaluation

Community engagement should be evaluated, just as any other aspect of the CTSA program, using clear and innovative metrics that can be applied uniformly and consistently at individual CTSAs and across the program. To date, a formal evaluation of the community engagement aspects of the CTSA Program as a whole has not been conducted. In recent stakeholder input provided by the Center for Community Health Education Research and Service and the CCPH, one respondent wrote that the lack of common metrics "hurts [the] CSTA [community engagement] programs' ability to measure, document, [and] communicate their value in a way that's understood by CTSA leadership locally and nationally" (Freeman and Seifer, 2013).

The CTSA Community Engagement Key Function Committee has a working group to develop a uniform set of outcomes and measurements. This working group identified examples of community-engaged research and developed a logic model to guide development of community engagement metrics (Eder et al., 2013) (see Figure 4-1). Additional possible

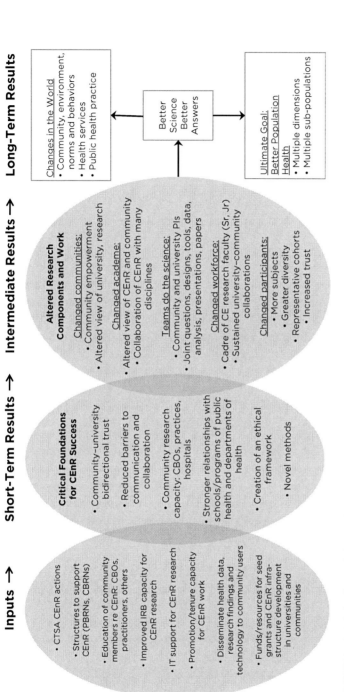

FIGURE 4-1 A logic model to guide community engagement metrics.

NOTE: CBOs = community-based organizations; CBRNs = community-based research networks; CE = community engagement; CEnR = community engagement research; IRB = institutional review board; IT = information technology; PBRNs = practice-based research networks.

SOURCE: Adapted with permission from Eder et al., 2013.

measures that have been suggested by researchers and community leaders include the following: extent of community partner integration into the research teams, documented research outcomes (e.g., community health improvements and outcomes, policy changes, successful translation), allocation of funds to community partners, and number of new and sustained community partnerships (Freeman and Seifer, 2013).

Opportunities and Next Steps

Because involving the community in the continuum of research is a new experience for many researchers, the CTSA Program and NCATS must provide clear guidance and leadership that effectively defines and communicates their goals and expectations. A number of barriers need to be overcome in order to establish effective community partnerships, including issues related to trust and respect, understanding the benefits and value of community engagement, challenges within academic cultures, a lack of clear expectations and protocols for engagement, and a lack of funding to compensate and provide training and education for community partners (Freeman and Seifer, 2013; Spofford et al., 2012). Models from individual CTSAs that have effectively incorporated members of the community throughout the research and translation process should be actively disseminated.

Although there is still much work to be done to integrate communities fully into all aspects of the CTSA Program, opportunities to embrace community engagement fully are increasing and are showing great promise. Electronic health records, social networking, and an increasingly active and sophisticated disease and health advocacy community can and should accelerate progress toward improvements in health status and reductions in health disparities. Partnerships with community engagement efforts sponsored by other NIH institutes and centers (e.g., the Research Centers in Minority Institutions program) offer potential for increasing the reach of CTSA's investments and strengthening the program's community engagement initiatives.

Throughout the study, the IOM committee heard overwhelming support for community engagement as an integral part of the CTSA program. An NIH working group on CTSA/NCATS integration, leaders of the CTSA Consortium, CTSA PIs, Congress, and a range of diverse stakeholders have all voiced support for the broad focus of the program, which encompasses the full spectrum of translational research, including community engagement (CTSA PIs, 2012; Katz et al., 2011; NCATS, 2012b; Pulley, 2013b; U.S. Congress, 2011). The IOM committee fully supports community engagement and involvement throughout the entire research process and believes that this program component is essential and needs to be preserved, nurtured, and expanded.

Community engagement should not be a stand-alone program requirement; it must be crosscutting and embedded in leadership, implementation, research, and communication strategies across all levels of the CTSA Program. Each CTSA site has unique strengths to build on, in addition to the opportunities afforded by the special interests, characteristics, and needs of the surrounding population or specific patient populations served. Inevitably, geographic and program diversity will lead to variations in the nature of community engagement from one site to another. But without clear incentives, metrics, and evaluation internally and from NCATS, the potential value in engaging community participants in the full range of activities—from basic discovery through patient outcomes—will not be realized.

Recommendation 6: *Ensure Community Engagement in All Phases of Research*

NCATS and the CTSA Program should ensure that patients, family members, health care providers, clinical researchers, and other community stakeholders are involved across the continuum of clinical and translational research. NCATS and the CTSA Program should

- **define community engagement broadly and use this definition consistently in RFAs and communications about the CTSA Program;**
- **ensure active and substantive community stakeholder participation in priority setting and decision making across all phases of clinical and translational research and in the leadership and governance of the CTSA Program;**
- **define and clearly communicate goals and expectations for community engagement at the individual CTSA level and across the program and ensure the broad dissemination of best practices in community engagement; and**
- **explore opportunities and incentives to engage a more diverse community.**

CHILD HEALTH RESEARCH

For too long, research examining the safety and efficacy of medications and other health interventions has focused on adults, and too little has been known about health- and development-related impacts of medications, devices, and preventive measures on children[3] (IOM, 2012b). Because of the paucity of pediatric-specific research, health care providers caring for children often use their own personal experiences in clinical practice, rather than published evidence, as the basis for treatment decisions (Kon, 2008). Thus, clinical and translational research is urgently needed in the area of child health. The IOM committee was specifically asked to look at child health research efforts in the CTSA Program and concluded that the program has placed an appropriate emphasis on accelerating clinical and translational research to improve child health.

The lack of pediatric studies results from a number of factors. Safety and ethical considerations for children participating in clinical trials are of primary concern, including the potential risks of exposing healthy volunteers to medications or other treatments that may have health or developmental side effects. Moreover, although some rare childhood diseases can be catastrophic, most children are healthy, which makes case finding for trials difficult. Additional challenges are the small market for pediatric drugs and devices, the smaller number of potential research participants, and variability among children because of age and developmental factors (IOM, 2012b). Further, because drugs and devices are often already approved for adults, they can be legally prescribed for children and may be widely used off label, before pediatric studies can be completed or even started (Portman, 2012).

Context and Background

Child health has been a focus of the CTSA Program. The NIH Reform Act of 2006 (Public Law 109-482) stipulated that independent

---

[3]In 1998 the NIH released policy guidelines for the inclusion of children in research (NIH, 1998). In the past two decades legislation aimed at increasing clinical trials involving children has included the Best Pharmaceuticals for Children Act (Public Law 107-109), the Pediatric Research Equity Act of 2003 (Public Law 108-155), and the Food and Drug Administration Safety and Innovation Act (Public Law 112-144). These initiatives support progress in pediatric clinical studies; however, empirical studies still need to be done in many areas.

funding and infrastructure for pediatric clinical research centers (formerly in the GCRCs) can be maintained. Subsequent to that legislation, the funding announcements for CTSAs have noted that applications can include a second principal investigator with authority for child health research and proposals for designating a separate budget for child health research (Huskins et al., 2012; NIH, 2009a). As of March 2013, 9 of the 61 CTSAs have a pediatrician as the principal investigator, and many have a designated pediatric or child health lead (Collier, 2013a). In addition, 53 CTSAs have some degree of partnership with children's hospitals (Collier, 2013a). Most CTSAs have pediatric researchers participating on the CTSA Consortium Child Health Oversight Committee (CC-CHOC).

The CC-CHOC was established in 2006 as one of the CTSA Consortium's leadership committees. Its mission and goals are to provide a national forum to identify collaborative opportunities for facilitating clinical and translational research on child health; to set priorities for the development of collaborative efforts and standard approaches; and to coordinate CTSA-wide efforts on child health research (CTSA Central, 2012a).

Several recent projects suggest the breadth of efforts spearheaded by CC-CHOC with participation by individual CTSAs:

- The Point Person Project works to overcome barriers that have hindered past efforts in pediatric research by ensuring that connections are made to respond to collaborative opportunities among industry, research networks, and investigators with relevant expertise for protocol and trial development and implementation (see Box 4-5).
- CC-CHOC is working toward the harmonization of policy and regulatory aspects of child health research, including efforts to standardize relevant terminology, case definitions, diagnostic criteria, and core outcome measures (CTSA Central, 2012a; Davis, 2012).
- CC-CHOC and participating CTSAs have developed a federated IRB model to provide a thorough and flexible IRB process to facilitate multisite pediatric clinical trials (CTSA Central, 2012a). For example, CC-CHOC has collaborated with the Rare Disease Clinical Research Network in the use of the centralized IRB model to test a treatment for infantile Pompe disease (CTSA Central, 2012a).

BOX 4-5
The Point Person Project

In an effort to increase the efficiency and response rate in multisite pediatric clinical trials, the CTSA Consortium Child Health Oversight Committee initiated the Point Person Project in 2012 (Davis, 2012). This program allows research sponsors, industry representatives, or individual developers to propose and explore interest in a range of child health research studies (CTSA Central, 2012b). A synopsis of the protocol is submitted to the CTSA Coordinating Center and reviewed by the CC-CHOC Operations Group, and, if approved, it is sent to the point person at each of the 55 CTSA sites with a pediatric program (Davis, 2012). The point person gives the synopsis link to investigators in their CTSA with related interests, and these investigators indicate whether they are interested, not interested, or need more information. The responses are entered into a central database, and those who are interested are invited to join a weekly conference call where the project is discussed with the sponsor (Children's National Medical Center CTSI, 2013). In the first 5 months of this program, 20 protocols were reviewed (Davis, 2012). In addition to facilitating collaborations and expediting the initiation of clinical trials, an additional benefit may be identifying and recruiting experts and collaborators for protocol development (Davis, 2012).

Interdisciplinary and multisite collaborations are particularly important for child health research. Multicenter studies are often necessary because of the small number of children who meet eligibility criteria for clinical trials. The developmental and physiological needs of children differ from those of adults and require the expertise of multiple disciplines in the design and conduct of clinical studies. One of CC-CHOC's short-term goals is to enhance interactions with child health research partners in the United States and globally. Efforts are under way to coordinate with NIH-related networks (e.g., Pediatric Trials Network), practice-based research and other research networks (e.g., the American Academy of Pediatrics' Pediatric Research in Office Settings Network, the Global Alliance for Pediatrics Therapeutics); and international networks (e.g., European Network of Pediatric Research at the European Medicines Agency) (Davis, 2012; Portman, 2012).

Safety and ethical considerations are of primary concern in child health research. CC-CHOC's Pediatric Research Ethics Workgroup has reviewed protocols submitted by CTSA pediatric investigators to determine trends in IRB decision making and is encouraging shared IRB approaches for multisite trials. The group also facilitates a pediatric research ethics consultation service to link research ethics consultants and pediatric investigators in order to strengthen requests for protocol approval (CTSA Central, 2013d).

CC-CHOC has ongoing efforts to develop evaluation metrics for child health research (Huskins et al., 2012). Further, it is surveying CTSAs regarding steps needed to enhance career pathways for child health investigators (Davis, 2012).

Opportunities and Next Steps

Leadership, Collaboration, and Evaluation in Child Health Research

The CTSA Program, through CC-CHOC, has made important steps in streamlining and accelerating clinical and translational research specific to the neglected area of child health. To strengthen these efforts, the IOM committee believes that the NCATS-CTSA Steering Committee should identify a relatively small number of CTSAs with established expertise and outstanding efforts in child health research as the leaders in this arena. Those designated CTSAs, in collaboration with CC-CHOC, would be charged with creating focused initiatives to develop key partnerships and collaborations across other CTSAs, and with the NIH and a variety of public and private sector research networks, including industry partners. The goal would be to strengthen the resources and leadership provided for child health research. These CTSAs would spearhead efforts to improve and accelerate clinical and translational research in child health, encourage research participation, and promote career pathways for child health investigators.

Identifying specific CTSAs to take the lead in child health research would not preclude other CTSAs from involvement in this area. Instead, the IOM committee hopes that such focused efforts would encourage and promote collaborations among CTSAs for multisite studies and other efforts. The committee also believes that the CTSAs should be engaged in a life-span approach that includes research on the transition from adolescence into adulthood.

As part of a learning health care system, child health researchers need to be sure that this area of investigation is well positioned to fully embrace the use of electronic health records for research purposes and to actively partner with PBRNs. Implementing these types of strategies will allow researchers to understand what is occurring in clinical practice and will allow pediatric health care providers, patients, and families to learn about new medications, therapeutics, and preventive measures.

The Involvement of Children, Parents, Family Members, and Community Organizations

Efforts to advance child health research need the active and direct involvement of patients, parents, family members, pediatric and family health care providers, and other community stakeholders in all phases of research. As a part of the team that guides clinical and translational research and encourages participation in this vital area, informed family and community participants will bring practical insights and dedicated commitment to setting research priorities, reviewing protocols, modifying trial designs, and ensuring adherence to research subjects' protection policies for clinical research involving children. Further, these groups can promote research participation. Recent study findings suggest that families know little about potential opportunities for participation in clinical research and often do not understand its potential benefits (Davis et al., 2013).

Conclusions and Recommendation

Research is needed on medications, devices, and preventive measures that specifically assesses their impact on children, whether they are targeted to specific diseases of children or are adult treatments used for pediatric patients. Primarily because of the much smaller population affected with pediatric diseases, many of these diseases are "orphan conditions," yet they can be life limiting or result in lifelong mental, physical, or developmental disabilities.

Because of the burden of these conditions, clinical and translational research is of special importance, and the IOM committee believes that the CTSA Program has placed an appropriate emphasis on accelerating clinical and translational research to improve child health. As a strong and vital part of the CTSA Program, the individual CTSAs and CC-CHOC have made important steps in this direction. The CTSA Program should continue its role in leading efforts to coordinate and advance child health research by building on the expertise of individual CTSAs and by ensuring that the CTSA Program continues to be a leader in developing and sustaining the collaborations necessary to move these efforts forward.

Recommendation 7: *Strengthen Clinical and Translational Research Relevant to Child Health*

NCATS should collaborate with CC-CHOC to strengthen clinical and translational research relevant to child health through efforts to

- identify and designate CTSAs with expertise in child health research as leaders in advancing clinical and translational research relevant to child health and as coordinators for CTSA programwide efforts and other collaborative efforts in this research; and
- promote and increase community engagement specific to child health by
  o raising awareness of the opportunities for children and families to participate in research efforts with clear information conveyed on the risks and potential benefits; and
  o involving parents, patients, and family members more fully at all stages of the research process, including identifying priorities and setting research agendas.

REFERENCES

Andrews, J. O., M. J. Cox, S. D. Newman, G. Gillenwater, G. Warner, J. A. Winkler, B. White, S. Wolf, R. Leite, M. E. Ford, and S. Slaughter. 2012. Training partnership dyads for community-based participatory research: Strategies and lessons learned from the community engaged scholars program. *Health Promotion Practice.*, October 22. Published online before print, doi: 10.1177/1524839912461273.

Brady, K. 2012. *CTSA strategic goal 4: Enhancing the health of our communities and the nation.* PowerPoint presented at Meeting 1: IOM Committee to Review the CTSA Program at NCATS, Washington, DC, October 29. http://www.iom.edu/~/media/Files/Activity%20Files/Research/ CTSAReview/2012-OCT-29/CTSA%20presentations/5-Brady%CTSA%20% 20SGC4%20slides%20for%20%20IOM.pdf (accessed March 25, 2013).

C3 (Chicago Consortium for Community Engagement). 2013. *Welcome to the C3 network.* http://c3ctsa.org (accessed March 25, 2013).

Carter-Edwards, L., J. L. Cook, M. A. McDonald, S. M. Weaver, K. Chukwuka, and M. M. Eder. 2013. Report on CTSA consortium use of the community engagement consulting service. *Clinical and Translational Science* 6(1):34–39.

Case Western Reserve University CTSC (Clinical and Translational Science Collaborative). 2012. *Clinical and Translational Science Collaborative: Key achievements, 2007–2012.* http://casemed.case.edu/ctsc/calendar/news/achievements.cfm (accessed March 25, 2013).

CCPH (Community-Campus Partnerships for Health). 2012a. *CCPH's response to NOT-TR-13-001 Request for Information: Enhancing community-engaged research through the CTSA Program.* http://depts.washington.edu/ccph/pdf_files/CCPH-RFI-Nov2012F3.pdf (accessed March 22, 2013).

———. 2012b. *Letter to Christopher P. Austin, Director of the National Center for Advancing Translational Sciences.* September 28. Submitted to the IOM Committee on October 12, 2012. Available by request through the National Academies' Public Access Records Office.

CDC and ATSDR (Centers for Disease Control and Prevention and Agency for Toxic Substances and Disease Registry). 1997. *Principles of community engagement.* http://www.cdc.gov/phppo/pce (accessed March 22, 2013).

Ceglia, L. 2013. *Presentation: KL2 award: One researcher's experience.* Remarks presented at Meeting 3: IOM Committee to Review the CTSA Program at NCATS, Washington, DC, January 24.

Children's National Medical Center CTSI (Clinical and Translational Science Institute). 2013. *Introducing the Point Person Project.* http://ctsicn.org/2013/01/introducing-the-point-person-project/ (accessed February 18, 2013).

Collier, E. 2013a. *Responses to committee questions.* Submitted to the IOM Committee on March 27. Available by request through the National Academies' Public Access Records Office.

———. 2013b. *Written comments regarding career development programs.* Submitted to the IOM Committee on April 2. Available by request through the National Academies' Public Access Records Office.

Community Partners (Community Recommendations Working Group of Community Partners). 2009. *Recommendations for community involvement in National Institute of Allergy and Infectious Diseases HIV/AIDS clinical trials research.* Washington, DC: National Institutes of Health. http://www.niaid.nih.gov/about/organization/daid/Networks/Documents/cabrecommendations.pdf (accessed March 22, 2013).

CTSA (Clinical and Translational Science Awards) Central. 2011. *Core competencies for clinical and translational research.* https://www.ctsacentral.org/education_and_career_development/core-competencies-clinical-and-translational-research (accessed March 22, 2013).

———. 2012a. *2012 Annual report: CTSA Consortium Child Health Oversight Committee.* https://www.ctsacentral.org/sites/default/files/documents/2012%20CC%20CHOC%20Annual%20Report.pdf (accessed March 20, 2013).

———. 2012b. *CC-CHOC Pediatric Point Person Project.* www.ctsacentral.org/documents/point-person-project (accessed April 22, 2013).

————. 2013a. *About the CTSA Consortium.* https://www.ctsacentral.org/about-us/ctsa (accessed February 13, 2013).

————. 2013b. *Chicago Consortium for Community Engagement.* http://www.ctsacentral.org/regional-consortia/chicago-consortium-community-engagement (accessed March 25, 2013).

————. 2013c. *Community Engagement Key Function Committee.* https://www.ctsacentral.org/committee/community-engagement (accessed March 25, 2013).

————. 2013d. *Pediatric research ethics consultation service.* https://www.ctsacentral.org/articles/pediatric-research-ethics-consultation-service (accessed March 20, 2013).

————. 2013e. *Strategic Goal Committee 2—training and career development of clinical/translational scientists.* https://www.ctsacentral.org/committee/sg2-training-and-career-development-clinicaltranslational-scientists (accessed March 11, 2013).

————. 2013f. *Strategic Goal Committee 4—enhancing the health of our communities and the nation.* https://www.ctsacentral.org/committee/sg4-enhancing-health-our-communities-and-nation (accessed March 25, 2013).

CTSA PIs (Principal Investigators). 2012. Preparedness of the CTSA's structural and scientific assets to support the mission of the National Center for Advancing Translational Sciences (NCATS). *Clinical and Translational Science* 5(2):121–129.

Davis, J. 2012. *The role of CC-CHOC in maternal child research.* PowerPoint presented at Meeting 2: IOM Committee to Review the CTSA Program at NCATS, Washington, DC, December 12. http://www.iom.edu/~/media/Files/Activity%20Files/Research/CTSAReview/2012-DEC-12/2-1%20%20Jonathan%20Davis.pdf (accessed February 18, 2013).

Davis, M. M., S. J. Clark, A. T. Butchart, D. C. Singer, T. P. Shanley, and D. S. Gipson. 2013. Public participation in, and awareness about, medical research opportunities in the era of clinical and translational research. *Clinical and Translational Science* 6(2):88–93.

Dieffenbach, C. 2011. *Community engagement in NIAID's HIV/AIDS clinical trials networks.* http://blog.aids.gov/2011/09/community-engagement-in-niaid%E2%80%99s-hivaids-clinical-trials-networks.html (accessed March 22, 2013).

Dolor, R. J., S. M. Greene, E. Thompson, L.-M. Baldwin, and A. V. Neale. 2011. Partnership-Driven Resources to Improve and Enhance Research (PRIMER): A survey of community-engaged researchers and creation of an online toolkit. *Clinical and Translational Science* 4(4):259–265.

Duke Center for Community Research. 2013. *Community Engagement Consultative Service (CECS).* https://www.dtmi.duke.edu/about-us/organization/duke-center-for-community-research/community-engagement-consultative-service-cecs (accessed March 25, 2013).

Eder, M., L. Carter-Edwards, T. C. Hurd, B. B. Rumala, N. Wallerstein. 2013. A logic model for community engagement within the CTSA Consortium: Can we measure what we model? *Academic Medicine* 88(10).

Edwards, K. 2013. *Using CTSAs to leverage change: New investigators, new science.* PowerPoint presented at Meeting 3: Committee to Review the CTSA Program at NCATS, Washington, DC, January 24. http://www.iom.edu/~/media/Files/Activity%20Files/Research/CTSAReview/2013-JAN-24/Kelly%20Edwards.pdf (accessed April 10, 2013).

Emmons, K. M. 2012. *Harvard Catalyst response to RFI NOT-TR-13-001.* Submitted to the IOM Committee on February 1, 2013. Available by request through the National Academies' Public Access Records Office.

ENACCT and CCPH (Education Network to Advance Cancer Clinical Trials and Community-Campus Partnerships for Health). 2008. *Communities as partners in cancer clinical trials: Changing research, practice and policy.* Silver Spring, MD: ENACCT. http://www.enacct.org/sites/default/files/CommunitiesAsPartners_Report_12_18_08_0.pdf (accessed March 22, 2013).

Fleming, M., E. L. Burnham, and W. C. Huskins. 2012. Mentoring translational science investigators. *JAMA* 308(19):1981–1982.

Freeman, E. R., and S. Seifer. 2013. *A Delphi process to solicit stakeholder feedback for the IOM Committee Review of the CTSA Program.* Submitted to the IOM Committee on March 3. Available by request through the National Academies' Public Access Records Office.

HANC (HIV/AIDS Network Coordination). 2013a. *Community Partners.* https://www.hanc.info/cp/Pages/default.aspx (accessed March 22, 2013).

———. 2013b. *The Legacy Project.* https://www.hanc.info/legacy/Pages/default.aspx (accessed March 22, 2013).

Harvard Medical School DCP (Office for Diversity Inclusion and Community Partnership). 2013. *The Harvard Catalyst Program for Faculty Development and Diversity. Program for college students: Summer Clinical and Translational Research Program.* http://www.mfdp.medp.med.harvard.edu/Catalyst/CollegeStudents.html (accessed April 1, 2013).

Hatcher, M. T., and R. M. Nicola. 2008. Building constituencies for public health. In *Public health administration: Principles for population-based management.* Vol. 2, edited by L. F. Novick, C. B. Morrow and G. P. Mays. Sudbury, MA: Jones and Bartlett. Pp. 443–458.

Healing of the Canoe. 2013. *The Healing of the Canoe Project.* http://healingofthecanoe.org (accessed March 19, 2013).

Hood, N. E., T. Brewer, R. Jackson, and M. E. Wewers. 2010. Survey of community engagement in NIH-funded research. *Clinical Translational Science* 3(1):19–22.

Horowitz, C. R., M. Robinson, and S. Seifer. 2009. Community-based participatory research from the margin to the mainstream: Are researchers prepared? *Circulation* 119(19):2633–2642.

HPS (Hermansky-Pudlak Syndrome) Network. 2013. *Hermansky-Pudlak Syndrome Network, Inc.* http://www.hpsnetwork.org (accessed March 18, 2013).

Huskins, W. C., K. Silet, A. M. Weber-Main, M. D. Begg, V. G. Fowler, J. Hamilton, and M. Fleming. 2011. Identifying and aligning expectations in a mentoring relationship. *Clinical and Translational Science* 4(6):439–447.

Huskins, W. C., C. D. Sullivan, J. Wang, M. Aitken, S. R. Alexander, L. G. Epstein, A. Hoberman, E. Neufeld, A. Philipps, T. P. Shanley, P. Szilagyi, M. Purucker, and S. L. Barkin. 2012. Tracking the impact of the National Institutes of Health Clinical and Translational Science Awards on child health research: Developing and evaluating a measurement strategy. *Pediatric Research* 71(5):619–624.

Indiana University CTSI (Clinical and Translational Sciences Institute). 2012. *CORUS (Community Research Utilities and Support): Working together to advance community engaged research.* https://ctsacorus.org/home (accessed March 25, 2013).

IOM (Institute of Medicine). 2012a. *Primary care and public health: Exploring integration to improve population health.* Washington, DC: The National Academies Press.

———. 2012b. *Safe and effective medicines for children: Pediatric studies conducted under the Best Pharmaceuticals for Children Act and the Pediatric Research Equity Act.* Washington, DC: The National Academies Press.

———. 2013. *Responses to public input questions regarding the CTSA Program at NCATS.* Submitted to the IOM Committee between December 17, 2012–March 1, 2013. Available by request through the National Academies' Public Access Records Office.

ITHS (Institute of Translational Health Sciences). 2013. *Education core.* www.iths.org/ED (accessed April 10, 2013).

Kagan, J. M., S. R. Rosas, R. L. Siskind, R. D. Campbell, D. Gondwe, D. Munroe, W. M. K. Trochim, and J. T. Schouten. 2012. Community-researcher partnerships at NIAID HIV/AIDS clinical trial sites: Insights for evaluation and enhancement. *Progress in Community Health Partnerships: Research, Education, and Action* 6(3):311–320.

Katz, S., J. Anderson, H. Auchincloss, J. Briggs, A. Guttmacher, K. Hudson, R. Hodes, W. Koroshetz, R. Ranganathan, G. Rodgers, and S. Shurin. 2011. *NIH CTSA/NCATS Integration Working Group recommendations.* http://www.ncats.nih.gov/files/recommendations.pdf (accessed April 8, 2013).

Kelley, M., K. Edwards, H. Starks, S. M. Fullerton, R. James, S. Goering, S. Holland, M. L. Disis, and W. Burke. 2012. Values in translation: How asking the right questions can move translational science toward greater health impact. *Clinical and Translational Science* 5(6):445–451.

Kon, A. A. 2008. Real pragmatism, kids, and the Clinical and Translational Science Award (CTSA). *American Journal of Bioethics* 8(4):45–47.

Lee, L. S., S. N. Pusek, W. T. McCormack, D. L. Helitzer, C. A. Martina, A. M. Dozier, J. S. Ahluwalia, L. S. Schwartz, L. M. McManus, B. D. Reynolds, E. N. Haynes, and D. M. Rubio. 2012. Clinical and translational scientist career success: Metrics for evaluation. *Clinical and Translational Science* 5(5):400–407.

Martinez, L. S., B. Russell, C. L. Rubin, L. K. Leslie, and D. Brugge. 2012. Clinical and translational research and community engagement: Implications for researcher capacity building. *Clinical and Translational Science* 5(4):329–332.

Meagher, E. A. 2011. Training translators in the PENN CTSA. *Clinical and Translational Science* 4(5):314–316.

Meyers, F. J., M. D. Begg, M. Fleming, and C. Merchant. 2012. Strengthening the career development of clinical translational scientist trainees: A consensus statement of the Clinical Translational Science Award (CTSA) research education and career development committees. *Clinical and Translational Science* 5(2):132–137.

Michener, L., J. Cook, S. M. Ahmed, M. A. Yonas, T. Coyne-Beasley, and S. Aguilar-Gaxiola. 2012. Aligning the goals of community-engaged research: Why and how academic health centers can successfully engage with communities to improve health. *Academic Medicine* 87(3):285–291.

Miyaoka, A., M. Spiegelman, K. Raue, and J. Frechtling. 2011. *Findings from the CTSA National Evaluation Education and Training Study.* Rockville, MD: Westat. https://ctsacentral.org/sites/default/files/documents/education TrainingReport_20111228.pdf (accessed April 1, 2013).

NCATS (National Center for Advancing Translational Sciences). 2012a. *FAQ about CTSA RFA-TR-12-006.* http://www.ncats.nigh.gov/research/cts/ctsa/ funding/faq/faq.html (accessed March 22, 2013).

———. 2012b. *Request for information: Enhancing the Clinical and Translational Science Awards Program.* http://www.ncats.nih.gov/files/ report-ctsa-rfi.pdf (accessed April 8, 2013).

———. 2013. *Scholar and research programs.* http://www.ncats.nih.gov/research/ cts/ctsa/training/programs/scholar-trainee.html (accessed March 11, 2013).

NIH (National Institutes of Health). 1998. *NIH policy and guidelines on the inclusion of children as participants in research involving human subjects.* http://grants.nih.gov/grants/guide/notice-files/not98-024.html (accessed March 20, 2013).

———. 2009a. *RFA-RM-09-004: Institutional Clinical and Translational Science Award (U54).* http://grants.nih.gov/grants/guide/rfa-files/RFA-RM-09-004.html (accessed March 22, 2013).

———. 2009b. *RFA-RM-09-019: Institutional Clinical and Translational Science Award (U54).* http://grants.nih.gov/grants/guide/rfa-files/RFA-RM-09-019.html (accessed March 22, 2013).

————. 2012a. Enhancing the health of our communities and the nation. Chapter 5. In *Progress Report 2009–2011 Clinical and Translational Science Awards: Foundations for accelerated discovery and efficient translation*. http://www.ncats.nih.gov/ctsa_2011/ch5.html (accessed April 1, 2013).

————. 2012b. *Request for information: Enhancing community-engaged research through the Clinical and Translational Science Awards (CTSA) Program.* http://grants.nih.gov/grants/guide/notice-files/NOT-TR-13-001.html (accessed March 22, 2013).

————. 2012c. *RFA-TR-12-006: Institutional Clinical and Translational Science Award (U54).* http://grants.nih.gov/grants/guide/rfa-files/rfa-tr-12-006.html (accessed February 13, 2013).

————. 2013a. *Increasing the diversity of the NIH-funded workforce: Program initiatives.* http://commonfund.nih.gov/diversity/initiatives.aspx (accessed March 11, 2013).

————. 2013b. *Notice of intent to publish a funding opportunity announcement for planning grants for the NIH National Research Mentoring Network.* http://grants.nih.gov/grants/guide/notice-files/NOT-RM-13-009.html (accessed April 30, 2013).

NIMHD (National Institute on Minority Health and Health Disparities). 2013. *NIMHD Research Centers in Minority Institutions Program.* http://www.nimhd.nih.gov/our_programs/research_centers.asp (accessed April 30, 2013).

Parsons, S. 2013. *Responses to committee questions.* Submitted to the IOM Committee on February 26. Available by request through the National Academies' Public Access Records Office.

Portman, R. 2012. *Children's health research: Role of the CTSA Program in pediatric drug development.* PowerPoint presented at Conference Call Meeting 2: IOM Committee to Review the CTSA Program at NCATS, Washington, DC, November 30. http://www.iom.edu/~/media/Files/Activity%20Files/Research/CTSAReview/2012-NOV-30/Ronald%20Portman.pdf (accesssed March 20, 2013).

Pulley, J. 2013a. *CTSA essays and worksheets. Submitted to the NIH CTSA/NCATS Integration Working Group, July 2011.* Submitted to the IOM Committee on January 7. Available by request through the National Academies' Public Access Records Office.

————. 2013b. *CTSA PI response to RFI NOT-TR-12-003.* Submitted to the IOM Committee on January 6. Available by request through the National Academies' Public Access Records Office.

PXE International. 2012. *PXE International Blood and Tissue Bank.* http://www.pxe.org/blood-tissue-bank (accessed March 22, 2013).

Research Toolkit. 2012. *Research toolkit: An active, growing library of resources for conducting health research.* http://www.researchtoolkit.org (accessed March 25, 2013).

Roberts, S. F., M. A. Fischhoff, S. A. Sakowski, and E. L. Feldman. 2012. Perspective: Transforming science into medicine: How clinician-scientists can build bridges across research's "valley of death." *Academic Medicine* 87(3):266–270.

Rubio, D. M., B. A. Primack, G. E. Switzer, C. L. Bryce, D. L. Seltzer, and W. N. Kapoor. 2011. A comprehensive career-success model for physician-scientists. *Academic Medicine* 86(12):1571–1576.

Seifer, S. D. 2013. *It's time to fully realize the potential of community engagement in the CTSA Program.* PowerPoint presented at Meeting 3: IOM Committee to Review the CTSA Program at NCATS, Washington, DC, January 24. http://www.iom.edu/~/media/Files/Activity%20Files/Research/CTSAReview/2013-JAN-24/Sarena%20Seifer.pdf (accessed March 22, 2013.

Shackelford, D. 2013. *Panel 1 presentation.* PowerPoint presented at Meeting 3: IOM Committee to Review the CTSA Program at NCATS, Washington, DC, January 24. http://www.iom.edu/~/media/Files/Activity%20Files/Research/CTSAReview/2013-JAN-24/David%20Shackelford.pdf (accessed April 2, 2013).

Silet, K. A., P. Asquith, and M. F. Fleming. 2010. A national survey of mentoring programs for KL2 scholars. *Clinical and Translational Science* 3(6):299–304.

Spofford, M., C. Wilkins, C. McKeever, and N. Williams. 2012. *Community representatives' involvement in CTSA activities: Summary.* Submitted to the IOM Committee on November 14. Available by request through the National Academies' Public Access Records Office.

Staley, K. 2009. *Exploring impact: Public involvement in NHS, public health and social care research.* Eastleigh, UK: Involve. http://www.invo.org.uk/wp-content/uploads/2011/11/Involve_Exploring_Impactfinal28.10.09.pdf (accessed March 22, 2013).

STSI (Scripps Translational Science Institute). 2013. *Community engagement.* http://www.stsiweb.org/index.php/community (accessed March 25, 2013).

Task Force on the Principles of Community Engagement (Clinical and Translational Science Awards Consortium Community Engagement Key Function Committee Task Force on the Principles of Community Engagement). 2011. *Principles of community engagement: Second edition.* NIH Publication No. 11-7782. http://www.atsdr.cdc.gov/communityengagement/pdf/PCE_Report_508_FINAL.pdf (accessed April 2, 2013).

Thomas, L. R., D. M. Donovan, and R. L. W. Sigo. 2010. Identifying community needs and resources in a native community: A research partnership in the Pacific Northwest. *International Journal of Mental Health and Addiction* 8(2):362–373.

Thomas, S. 2013. *Presentation: Roundtable discussion: Future directions for the mission and goals of the CTSA Program.* PowerPoint presented at Meeting 3: Committee to Review the CTSA Program at NCATS, Washington, DC, January 24.

Tillman, R. E., S. Jang, Z. Abedin, B. F. Richards, B. Spaeth-Rublee, and H. A. Pincus. 2013. Policies, activities, and structures supporting research monitoring: A national survey of academic health centers with clinical and translational science awards. *Academic Medicine* 88(1):90–96.

University of California, San Francisco CTSI (Clinical and Translational Science Institute). 2013. *Mentor development program: Course materials.* http://accelerate.ucsf.edu/training/mdp-materials (accessed April 10, 2013).

University of Cincinnati CCTST (Center for Clinical and Translational Science and Training). 2013. *University of Cincinnati: Center for Clinical and Translational Science and Training.* http://cctst.uc.edu/programs/community/cli (accessed March 25, 2013).

University of Iowa ICTS (Institute for Clinical and Translational Science). 2013. *Virtual University.* https://virtualu2.icts.uiowa.edu (accessed March 11, 2013).

University of Pennsylvania ITMAT (Institute for Translational Medicine and Therapeutics). 2013. *CTSA ITMAT education.* http://www.itmat.upenn.edu/ctsa/ctsa_education.shtml (accessed March 11, 2013).

University of Rochester CTSI (Clinical and Translational Science Institute). 2013. *All courses.* https://research.urmc.rochester.edu/ncerp/search (accessed March 11, 2013).

U.S. Congress, House of Representatives. 2011. *Military Constructions and Veterans Affairs and Related Agencies Appropriations Act: Conference report to accompany HR 2055.* 112th Cong., 1st sess. http://www.gpo.gov/fdsys/pkg/CRPT-112hrpt331/pdf/CRPT-112hrpt331.pdf (accessed May 6, 2013).

Van Hartesveldt, C., J. Giordan, and IGERT(Integrative Graduate Educate and Research Traineeship) Program Directors. 2008. *Impact of transformative interdisciplinary research and graduate education on academic institutions.* http://www.nsf.gov/pubs/2009/nsf0933/igert_workshop08.pdf (accessed April 10, 2013).

Woolf, S. H. 2008. The meaning of translational research and why it matters. *Journal of the American Medical Association* 299(2):211–213.

Yarborough, M., K. Edwards, P. Espinoza, G. Geller, A. Sarwal, R. R. Sharp, and P. Spicer. 2012. Relationships hold the key to trustworthy and productive translational science: Recommendations for expanding community engagement in biomedical research. *Clinical and Translational Science*, January 14. Published online before print, doi: 10.1111/cts.12022.

Young, L. R., R. Pasula, P. M. Gulleman, G. H. Deutsch, and F. X. McCormack. 2007. Susceptibility of Hermansky-Pudlak mice to bleomycin-induced type II cell apoptosis and fibrosis. *American Journal of Respiratory Cell and Molecular Biology* 37(3):67–74.

5

Conclusion: Opportunities for Action

In its first 7 years, the Clinical and Translational Science Awards (CTSA) Program has served as a foundation and catalyst for clinical and translational research at 61 academic health centers and other institutions across the United States. With the ultimate goal of improving human health, the CTSA Program now has the opportunity to propel clinical and translational research efforts forward rapidly. To move to CTSA 2.0, the CTSA Program can build on its foundation, draw on the creativity and dedication of CTSA principal investigators, researchers, and staff; use the ever-expanding capabilities of informatics and other technologies; share data and research support tools as openly and freely as possible; and fully engage new cadres of researchers focused on team-based science. Looking forward, the committee has identified four key opportunities for action:

- adopt and sustain active program leadership;
- engage in substantive and productive collaborations;
- develop and widely disseminate innovative research resources; and
- build on initial successes in training and education, community engagement, and child health research.

The next steps can be accomplished at multiple levels:

- The National Center for Advancing Translational Sciences (NCATS) has responsibilities to increase its leadership presence for the CTSA Program. This effort will require working with all program components to set goals and provide incentives and direction in order to move to a fully integrated network focused on accelerating clinical and translational research.

- The multiple components of the CTSA Program should work together under the direction of the recommended NCATS-CTSA Steering Committee to streamline the consortium structure, engage all individual CTSAs in meeting strategic goals and objectives, and use the Coordinating Center to share and implement best practices.
- Individual CTSAs can bring their creativity and institutional strengths and their local collaborations to bear on removing barriers and solving the larger challenges of clinical and translational research. By engaging their local communities and building on their expertise, individual CTSAs can be active hubs within the larger CTSA Program network.
- Community organizations and individuals, practice-based research networks, the HMO Research Network, industry partners, other NIH institutes and centers, and other potential collaborators can explore the opportunities that the CTSA Program provides and can push NCATS and individual CTSAs to engage in truly collaborative ventures focused on facilitating and accelerating clinical and translational research.

In conclusion, the Institute of Medicine (IOM) committee believes that the CTSA Program should be the national leader for advancing innovative and transformative clinical and translational research to improve human health. To achieve this, the CTSA Program should reshape its goals to reflect its new location within NCATS; build on the work of individual CTSAs to provide institutional leadership; focus on team-based education and training; and establish a national network that will accelerate the development of new diagnostics, therapeutics, and preventive interventions and, at the same time, drive innovation in clinical and translational research methods, processes, tools, and resources.

Because the CTSA Program is not disease specific in its orientation, strong collaborations must be forged across disciplinary units within individual CTSA institutions and with other NIH institutes and centers, as well as with other government funders, industry, philanthropies, and community organizations.

The CTSA Program should continue to lead efforts in expanding and diversifying the research workforce and to coordinate and advance child health by streamlining and building on the expertise of individual CTSAs. In all these efforts, community engagement is essential.

The contributions of individual CTSAs and the CTSA Program are vital to the clinical and translational research enterprise, and the nation's health can benefit greatly from strengthening their efforts.

A

Data Sources and Methods

The Institute of Medicine (IOM) Committee to Review the Clinical and Translational Science Awards (CTSA) Program at the National Center for Advancing Translational Sciences (NCATS) was tasked with providing an independent appraisal of the CTSA Program. The specific goals of this congressionally requested review were to assess the CTSA Program's mission and goals and to explore the contributions of the CTSA Program in accelerating the development of new therapeutics, in facilitating disease-specific research and children's health research, and in enhancing the integration of programs funded by the National Institutes of Health (NIH) institutes and centers. In conducting its work and responding to the statement of task, the IOM committee reviewed information that was collected from a variety of sources, including scientific literature, previous evaluations and progress reports, open-session meetings and conference calls, public testimony and input, and other publicly available resources.

COMMITTEE EXPERTISE

The study committee comprised 13 individuals with expertise in community outreach and engagement, public health and health policy, bioethics, education and training, pharmaceutical research and development, program evaluation, clinical and biomedical research, and child health research, along the full continuum of clinical and translation research. Appendix B provides biographical sketches of each of the committee members. The committee's expertise was supplemented by the knowledge and insights of a number of experts who presented research during open-session meetings and conference calls.

OPEN-SESSION MEETINGS, CONFERENCE CALLS, AND PUBLIC INPUT

Between October 2012 and February 2013, the committee convened three open-session meetings and four open-session conference calls (Boxes A-1 to A-7). The committee's first meeting in October was held remotely via conference call because of weather conditions associated with Hurricane Sandy. Over the course of the study, the committee also held a number of closed-session conference calls and a closed-session meeting in March 2013 to conclude its deliberations. The open-session meetings and calls allowed the committee to hear from a wide range of stakeholders, including a number of CTSA principal investigators and researchers, members of the NCATS and NIH leadership, community and patient advocacy organizations, industry partners and representatives, and thought leaders and researchers in the clinical and translational sciences arena who were not connected to the CTSA Program.

Each of the open-session meetings included a public comment period that allowed the committee to hear from other researchers, stakeholders, and members of the public. Because of budget constraints, all of the open-session meetings were held in Washington, DC. To provide additional opportunities for public input by individuals who were unable to travel to the meetings or participate by conference call, the committee used an online public input tool with questions to guide further testimony and input. A link to the public input tool was made available on the IOM's website from December 2012 through March 2013. The NCATS and IOM study listservs were used to notify stakeholders and the public about the opportunity to provide additional input to the committee's work and the availability of the online tool. The list of questions included in the public input tool can be found in Box A-8. During the 3 months that the tool was available, 27 individuals submitted responses to the questions. This input was catalogued in the study's public access file and is available by request through the National Academies' Public Access Records Office. The committee also reviewed input submitted through its e-mail address, CTSAReview@nas.edu, throughout the duration of the study.

INFORMATION GATHERING AND DOCUMENT REVIEW

In addition to information that was gathered during the open-session meetings and conference calls, the committee conducted a review of the available scientific literature with a focus on areas related to the CTSA Program and its work in clinical and translational sciences, training and education, community engagement, and child health research. The committee also reviewed previous evaluations of the CTSA Program, including the reports from the 3-year Westat evaluation and the evaluation of the administration of the CTSA Program under the NIH's National Center for Research Resources that was conducted by the Department of Health and Human Services' Office of the Inspector General; progress reports developed by the CTSA Consortium committees and the NIH; responses to the NIH's requests for information related to the CTSA Program; a wealth of information provided by NCATS, a range of CTSA Consortium committees, and stakeholder groups; and results and recommendations from other working groups and stakeholder meetings that have considered the future directions of the CTSA Program. Any information that was provided to the committee from outside sources was catalogued in the study's public access file and is available by request through the National Academies' Public Access Records Office.

BOX A-1
Committee to Review the Clinical and Translational Science
Awards Program at the National Center for Advancing
Translational Sciences
500 Fifth Street, NW
Washington, DC

Monday, October 29, 2012

Agenda

9:30 - 9:45	**Welcome and Introductions** *Alan Leshner*, Committee Chair *Sharon Terry*, Committee Vice-Chair
9:45 - 11:30	**Charge to the Committee and Discussion of Statement of Task** *Chris Austin*, Director, NCATS, NIH *Josie Briggs*, Acting Director, Division of Clinical Innovation, NCATS, NIH

11:30 - 12:30	Lunch Break

| 12:30 - 2:30 | **Overview of CTSA Committees and Strategic Goals**
CTSA Consortium Steering and Executive Committees
Bradley Evanoff, Washington University

Goal 1: National Clinical and Translational Research Capability
Clay Johnston, University of California, San Francisco

Goal 2: Training and Career Development of Clinical/Translational Scientists
Robert Toto, University of Texas Southwestern Medical Center

Goal 3: Consortium-Wide Collaborations
Anantha Shekhar, Indiana University

Goal 4: Health of Our Communities and the Nation
Kathleen Brady, Medical University of South Carolina

Goal 5: Advance T1 Translational Research
Nora Disis, University of Washington

Q&A with Panelists and Committee Discussion |

| 2:30 - 2:45 | **Break** |

| 2:45 - 4:45 | **Enhancing Integration: CTSAs and NIH Institutes and Centers**

National Cancer Institute
Linda Weiss, Director, Office of Cancer Centers, NCI, NIH
National Heart, Lung, and Blood Institute
Susan Shurin, Deputy Director, NHLBI, NIH
National Institute of Allergy and Infectious Diseases
Hugh Auchincloss, Deputy Director, NIAID, NIH
National Institute of Diabetes and Digestive and Kidney Diseases
Gregory G. Germino, Deputy Director, NIDDK, NIH
National Institute of Neurological Disorders and Stroke
Walter J. Koroshetz, Deputy Director, NINDS, NIH

Q&A with Panelists and Committee Discussion |

| 4:45 | **Public Comment Period** |

| 5:00 | **Adjourn** |

BOX A-2
Committee to Review the Clinical and Translational Science
Awards Program at the National Center
for Advancing Translational Sciences

Conference Call - November 19, 2012
11 a.m. to Noon (Eastern)

Agenda

11:00 - 12:00   Open Session
                  • *Nora Volkow*, NIDA
                  • *Steve Katz*, NIAMS

BOX A-3
Committee to Review the Clinical and Translational Science Awards Program
at the National Center
for Advancing Translational Sciences

Conference Call - November 30, 2012
10:30 a.m. to Noon (Eastern)

Agenda

10:30 - 12:00   Open Session
                  • *Steve Hirschfield*, NICHD
                  • *Dianne Murphy*, FDA
                  • *Charles Thompson*, Pfizer Inc.
                  • *Ron Portman*, Bristol-Meyers Squibb
                  • *Phil Pizzo*, Stanford University

BOX A-4
Committee to Review the Clinical and Translational
Science Awards Program at the National Center
for Advancing Translational Sciences

National Academy of Sciences Building
2101 Constitution Avenue, NW
Washington, DC

Wednesday, December 12, 2012

Agenda

8:00 - 8:05   Welcome and Opening Remarks
                  Alan Leshner, Chair

8:05 - 8:20	**CTSA Overview - Goals of the Program** *Tom Insel*, National Institute of Mental Health, NIH
8:20 - 9:50	**Panel 1: Translation of Basic Science to Human Studies: Advancing T1 and T2 Research** Facilitator: *Cliff Rosen*

8:20 - 8:25	Panel Introductions
8:25 - 8:35	CTSA Perspective *Garret FitzGerald*, University of Pennsylvania
8:35 - 8:45	CTSA Perspective *Sundeep Khosla*, Mayo Clinic
8:45 - 8:55	Community Perspective *Bernard Ewigman*, University of Chicago
8:55 - 9:05	Industry Perspective *Jacqueline B. Fine*, Merck Research Laboratories
9:05 - 9:50	Discussion with the Committee

9:50 - 10:00	**Break**
10:00 - 11:30	**Panel 2: Children's Health Research: Role of the CTSA Program** Facilitators: *Meg McCabe and Phyllis Dennery*

10:00 - 10:05	Panel Introductions
10:05 - 10:15	CTSA Consortium Child Health Oversight Committee *Jonathan Davis*, Tufts University
10:15 - 10:25	CTSA Perspective *Margaret Grey*, Yale School of Nursing
10:25 - 10:35	CTSA Perspective *Terence Flotte*, University of Massachusetts
10:35 - 10:45	Community Perspective *Susan Weiner*, Children's Cause for Cancer Advocacy
10:45 - 11:30	Discussion with the Committee

11:45 - 12:30	**Lunch**
12:30 - 1:45	**Panel 3: Collaborations Across CTSAs: Current Status and Future Plans** Facilitator: *Sue Curry*

12:30 - 12:35	Panel Introductions

	12:35 - 12:45	CTSA Coordinating Center (C4) Overview *Gordon Bernard*, Vanderbilt University
	12:45 - 12:55	Collaborations on Informatics *Paul Harris*, Vanderbilt University
	12:55 - 1:05	CTSA Perspective *Marc Drezner*, University of Wisconsin
	1:05 - 1:15	Community Perspective *Mickey Eder*, Access Community Health Network, Chicago
	1:15 - 1:45	Discussion with the Committee

1:45 - 3:00   **Panel 4: Evaluating the CTSA Program**
Facilitator: *Robin Kelley*

	1:45 - 1:50	Panel Introductions
	1:50 - 2:00	Westat Evaluations *Joy Frechtling*, Westat
	2:00 - 2:10	NCATS Request for Information *Josie Briggs*, NCATS, NIH
	2:10 - 2:20	NCATS/CTSA Integration Working Group *Steve Katz*, NIAMS, NIH
	2:20 - 2:30	Evaluating Large Scale Programs—Frameworks and Considerations *David Chavis*, Community Science
	2:30 - 3:00	Discussion with the Committee

3:00 - 3:15   **Break**

3:15 - 4:45   **Panel 5: Roundtable Discussion: Future Directions for the Mission and Goals of the CTSA Program**

	3:15 - 3:20	Roundtable Introductions
	3:20 - 4:00	Opening Comments on the CTSA Program *Tachi Yamada*, Takeda Pharmaceuticals (via conference call) *Wylie Burke*, University of Washington (via conference call) *John Adams*, University of California, Los Angeles
	4:00 - 4:45	Roundtable and Committee Discussion

4:45 - 5:30   **Public Comment Period**

5:30   **Adjourn**

BOX A-5

**Committee to Review the Clinical and Translational
Science Awards Program at the National Center
for Advancing Translational Sciences**

20F Conference Center
20 F Street, NW
Washington, DC

Thursday, January 24, 2013

Agenda

8:00 - 8:05   **Welcome and Opening Remarks**
                 Alan Leshner, Chair

8:05 - 8:45   Opening Speaker
                 Chris Austin, NCATS

8:45 - 10:10   **Panel 1: Training and Education**
                 Facilitator: *Cliff Rosen*

                 8:45 - 8:50   Panel Introductions
                 8:50 - 9:30   Panel Presentations
                                  David Shackelford, University of California
                                  Los Angeles
                                  Lisa Ceglia, Tufts University
                                  Kelly Edwards, University of Washington
                                  Cynthia Morris, Oregon Health and
                                  Science University
                 9:30 - 10:10   Discussion with the Committee

10:10 - 10:20   **Break**

10:20 - 11:45   **Panel 2: Engaging Community Organizations and Patient
                          Advocacy Groups**
                 Facilitators: *Sharon Terry and Susan Axelrod*

                 10:20 - 10:25   Panel Introductions
                 10:25 - 11:05   Panel Presentations
                                  Donna Appell, Hermansky-Pudlak
                                  Syndrome Network Inc.
                                  Bray Patrick-Lake, Clinical Trials
                                  Transformation Initiative

		Sarena Seifer, Community-Campus Partnerships for Health
		Joan Reede, Harvard University
	11:05 - 11:45	Discussion with the Committee

11:45 - 12:30	**Lunch Break**

12:30 - 2:00   **Panel 3   Advancing Research on Clinical Practice and Population Health: T3 and T4 Research**
Facilitator: *Ann Bonham*

	12:30 - 12:35	Panel Introductions
	12:35 - 1:15	Panel Presentations
		Lloyd Michener, Duke University
		Joe Selby, PCORI (Patient-Centered Outcomes Research Institute)
		Leonard Sacks, FDA
		John Steiner, Kaiser Permanente Colorado
	1:15 - 2:00	Discussion with the Committee

2:00 - 3:15   **Panel 4:   Future Directions for Using CTSA Programs and Resources**
Facilitator: *Ralph Horwitz*

	2:00 - 2:05	Panel Introductions
	2:05 - 2:35	Panel Presentations
		Robert Califf, Duke University
		Martha Curley, University of Pennsylvania
		Edith Parker, University of Iowa
	2:35 - 3:15	Discussion with the Committee

3:15 - 3:30	**Break**

3:30 - 5:00   **Panel 5:   Roundtable Discussion: Future Directions for the Mission and Goals of the CTSA Program**
Facilitator: *Edith Perez*

	3:30 - 3:35	Roundtable Introductions
	3:35 - 4:05	Opening Comments on the CTSA Program
		Morrie Schambelan, University of California, San Francisco
		Stephen Thomas, University of Maryland
		Gigi Hirsch, Massachusetts Institute of Technology

4:05 - 5:00	Roundtable and Committee Discussion
5:00 - 5:30	**Public Comment Period**
5:30	**Adjourn**

BOX A-6
Committee to Review the Clinical and Translational Science Awards Program at the National Center for Advancing Translational Sciences

Conference Call - January 30, 2013
12:30 to 2:00 p.m. (Eastern)

Agenda

12:30 - 2:00	**Open Session**	
	12:35 - 12:40	Welcoming Remarks *Alan Leshner*, Committee Chair
	12:40 - 12:50	*Petra Kaufmann*, NINDS, NIH
	12:50 - 1:00	Committee Q&A
	1:00 - 1:20	Discussion with *Francis Collins*, NIH
	1:20 - 1:30	*Eric Topol*, Scripps Research Institute
	1:30 - 2:00	Committee Q&A

BOX A-7
Committee to Review the Clinical and Translational Science Awards Program at the National Center for Advancing Translational Sciences

Conference Call - February 27, 2013
3:30 to 4:30 p.m. (Eastern)

Agenda

3:30 - 4:30	**Open Session** Discussion with *Chris Austin*, Director of NCATS

BOX A-8
Public Input Questions

Mission
- Is the mission of the CTSA Program clear and appropriate for defining the success of the program and for supporting the mission of NCATS?
- Is the scope of the mission realistic given the available resources, support, and infrastructure?
- Is the mission being disseminated adequately? Are potential stakeholders aware of the resources available through the CTSA Program, and are there barriers to the use of those resources?

Strategic Goals
- Are the strategic goals of the CTSA Program clear and appropriate? Do they clarify the purpose and mission of the CTSA Program?
- Are the strategic goals realistic given the available resources, support, and infrastructure?
- Are the strategic goals being disseminated adequately?
- Do you have suggestions for refocusing and revising the strategic goals of the CTSA Program?

Role of the CTSA
- Since the inception of the CTSA Program, have the CTSA institutions, individually and collectively, played an appropriate and adequate role in: (please check the boxes where you believe the CTSA Program has played an adequate and appropriate role)
  - accelerating the development of new therapeutics
  - facilitating disease-specific research
  - facilitating children's health and pediatric research
  - enhancing the integration of research funded by the NIH institutes and centers
  - involving and interacting with community organizations and patient advocacy groups?
- Could the mission and strategic goals be improved to address these issues? If so, how should they be improved?

Continuum of Research
- Please comment on the balance of CTSA Program efforts across the continuum of research from first-phase studies in humans to clinical trials to population-based research on health outcomes and comparative effectiveness.
- Does the balance need to shift? Why or why not?

Successes, Challenges, and Future Directions
- What do you see as successes, challenges, and future directions of the CTSA Program?

Additional Comments

B

Committee Biographical Sketches

Alan I. Leshner, Ph.D. (*Chair*), is chief executive officer of the American Association for the Advancement of Science (AAAS) and executive publisher of its journal, *Science*. Previously, Dr. Leshner served as director of the National Institute on Drug Abuse at the National Institutes of Health (NIH) and as deputy director and acting director of the National Institute of Mental Health. Before that, he held a variety of senior positions at the National Science Foundation. Dr. Leshner began his career at Bucknell University, where he was professor of psychology. Dr. Leshner is an elected member of the Institute of Medicine (IOM) of the National Academies of Science and a fellow of AAAS, the National Academy of Public Administration, and the American Academy of Arts and Sciences. He was appointed by President George W. Bush to the National Science Board and reappointed by President Obama. He received an A.B. in psychology from Franklin and Marshall College and his M.S. and Ph.D. in physiological psychology from Rutgers University. Dr. Leshner has been awarded six honorary doctor of science degrees.

Sharon F. Terry, M.A. (*Vice-Chair*), is president and chief executive officer of the Genetic Alliance, a network of more than 10,000 organizations, of which 1,200 are disease advocacy organizations. Genetic Alliance aims to improve health through the authentic engagement of communities and individuals. It also works to develop innovative solutions through novel partnerships, connecting consumers to smart services. Ms. Terry is also the founding chief executive officer of PXE International, a research advocacy organization for the genetic condition pseudoxanthoma elasticum (PXE). As codiscoverer of the gene associated with PXE, she holds the patent for ABCC6 and has assigned her rights to the foundation. She developed a diagnostic test and conducts clinical trials. Ms. Terry is also a cofounder of the Genetic Alliance Registry and Biobank. She is the author of more than 90 peer-reviewed articles. In her focus on consumer participation in genetics research, services, and policy, she serves in a leadership role on many of the major international and national organizations, including the IOM's Board on Health Sciences Policy, the IOM Roundtable on Translating Genomic-Based Research for Health, the board of the National Coalition for Health Professional Education in Genetics, the International Rare Disease Research Consortium Interim Executive Committee, and the newly formed Invoke Health! She is on the editorial boards of several journals and was instrumental in the passage of the Genetic Information Nondiscrimination Act. Among her awards are an honorary doctorate from Iona College in 2005 for her work in community engagement, the first Patient Service Award from the University of North Carolina's Institute for Pharmacogenomics and Individualized Therapy in 2007, the Research!America Distinguished Organization Advocacy Award in 2009, and the Clinical Research Forum and Foundation's Annual Award for Leadership in Public Advocacy in 2011. She is currently an Ashoka Fellow.

Susan Axelrod is chair and founder of Citizens United for Research in Epilepsy (CURE). In 1998 Ms. Axelrod and other mothers joined forces to raise funds to invest in the search for a cure for epilepsy. She has brought national and international media exposure to epilepsy, appearing on television news programs as well as special featured segments. Both *Parade* and *Newsweek* magazine articles have featured Ms. Axelrod and her family's journey with epilepsy. Ms. Axelrod has received numerous awards and honors for her leadership from Research!America, the Child Neurology Foundation, and the American Epilepsy Society, among others. She has spoken and served as a panelist at international conferences focused on medical philanthropy and advances and has served on the NIH's National Advisory Neurological Disorders and Stroke Council and as a reviewer for the Medical Research Program within the Department of Defense. Ms. Axelrod received a master's degree in business administration from the University of Chicago.

Enriqueta C. Bond, Ph.D., served from 1994 to 2008 as the first full-time president of the Burroughs Wellcome Fund (BWF), a private, independent foundation dedicated to advancing the medical sciences by supporting research and other scientific and educational activities. During her presidency Dr. Bond guided BWF in its transition from a corporate to a private foundation. Prior to joining the BWF, Dr. Bond served as the executive officer for the IOM. In 1997 she was elected as a member of the IOM. In 2004 she was elected as a fellow to the AAAS for her distinguished contributions to the study and analysis of policy for the advancement of the health sciences. Dr. Bond is chairman of the National Research Council's Board on African Science Academy Development and a member of the Forum on Microbial Threats. She is a past member of the National Academies' Report Review Committee as well as numerous other study committees. Dr. Bond is the recipient of numerous honors, including the 2008 Order of the Long Leaf Pine award from the state of North Carolina. The highest honor the governor can bestow on a citizen, this award was given to Dr. Bond for her efforts to improve science education for the children of North Carolina. She has also received the IOM Walsh McDermott Medal in recognition of distinguished service to the National Academies and received the National Academy of Sciences Professional Staff Award. She received her bachelor's degree from Wellesley College, her M.A. from the University of Virginia, and her Ph.D. in molecular biology and biochemical genetics from Georgetown University.

Ann C. Bonham, Ph.D., is chief scientific officer of the Association of American Medical Colleges and directs an array of programs supporting all aspects of research and research training. She serves on the IOM Forum on Drug Discovery, Development, and Translation and on the Department of Veterans Affairs National Research Advisory Council. Dr. Bonham was awarded the 2012 Distinguished Alumni Award for Achievement from the University of Iowa Carver School of Medicine and was the 2010 recipient of the Society for Executive Leadership in Academic Medicine International Award for Excellence. Prior to joining the association, Dr. Bonham served as executive associate dean for academic affairs and professor of pharmacology and internal medicine at the University of California (UC), Davis, School of Medicine. Dr. Bonham, a member of the UC Davis faculty for almost 20 years, played a major role in UC Davis's expansion of translational sciences and the School of Medicine's emphasis on combining research, education, and mentoring as interwoven and inseparable missions. As executive associate dean, Dr. Bonham oversaw the School of Medicine's research, undergraduate medical education, and faculty academic programs. She previously served as chair of the Department of Pharmacology. She also served as vice-chair of research for the Department of Internal Medicine and chief of the Division of Cardiovascular Medicine. She was twice awarded the UC Davis Kaiser Award for Excellence in Teaching Science Basic to Medicine and was honored with the American Medical Women's Association Gender Equity Award for providing a gender-fair environment for the education and training of women physicians. She has been recognized for her role in initiating training opportunities, mentoring fellows and students who have accepted positions in academics and industry, bringing together investigators to work in teams toward common goals, and fostering collaborations with faculty and department chairs across disciplines.

Susan J. Curry, Ph.D., is dean of the University of Iowa College of Public Health. She is recognized internationally for expertise in behavioral science and translation of research findings into health policy. Her extensive research on tobacco includes studies of motivations to quit smoking, randomized trials of promising smoking cessation and prevention interventions, evaluations of the use and cost-effectiveness of tobacco cessation treatments under different health insurance plans, and health care costs and utilization associated with tobacco cessation. Dr. Curry's research also encompasses studies of dietary change, modification of risky drinking patterns, and methods of increasing compliance with recommended cancer screening. She has served as a principal investigator or coinvestigator on 30 grants funded by the NIH, the Centers for Disease Control and Prevention, and major foundations. Dr. Curry has served on numerous national advisory boards, including the National Cancer Policy Board of the IOM, the Tobacco Cessation Consortium of the American Academy of Pediatrics, and the Subcommittee on Cessation of the Interagency Committee on Smoking and Health. She currently serves on the board of directors for the American Legacy Foundation and is a member of the U.S. Preventive Services Task Force. She received her Ph.D. in psychology from the University of New Hampshire. In 2010 Dr. Curry was elected a member of the IOM.

Phyllis A. Dennery, M.D., FAAP, is professor of pediatrics at the University of Pennsylvania and the Werner and Gertrude Henle Chair in Pediatrics at the Children's Hospital of Philadelphia. She serves as the chief of the Division of Neonatology and Newborn Services at the Children's Hospital of Philadelphia and the University of Pennsylvania Health System, where she oversees more than 280 intensive-care beds as well as more than 80 practitioners and 18 trainees. Dr. Dennery is the recipient of many awards and honors, including the Andrew Mellon Fellowship, the Ross Young Investigator Award from the Western Society of Pediatrics, the Alfred Stengel Health System Champion Award from the University of Pennsylvania, an honorary doctorate of science from Ursinus College, and the Mentor of the Year Award from the Eastern Society for Pediatric Research, among others. She has been listed as a "Top Doctor" in *U.S. News & World Report* and in *Philadelphia Magazine.* Dr. Dennery is also an active member of many professional and scientific societies. She served as the president of the Society for Pediatric Research and is currently the president of the International Pediatric Research Foundation. In addition to being the author of more than 100 publications, Dr. Dennery is associate editor for *Free Radicals in Biology and Medicine* and *Pediatrics* and a grant reviewer for the NIH. Her area of basic science research is the regulation of lung gene expression in oxidative stress, in particular the role of heme oxygenase, the rate-limiting enzyme in bilirubin production. Her clinical interests are in neonatal jaundice, bronchopulmonary dysplasia, and the long-term consequences of prematurity.

Ralph I. Horwitz, M.D., MACP, is senior vice-president for clinical evaluation sciences at GlaxoSmithKline (GSK) and Harold H. Hines Jr. Professor Emeritus of Medicine and Epidemiology at Yale University. Dr. Horwitz trained in internal medicine at institutions (Royal Victoria Hospital of McGill University and the Massachusetts General Hospital) where science and clinical medicine were strongly connected. These experiences as a resident stimulated a deep interest in clinical research training, which Dr. Horwitz pursued as a fellow in the Robert Wood Johnson Clinical Scholars Program at Yale under the direction of Alvan R. Feinstein. He joined the Yale faculty in 1978 and remained there for 25 years as codirector of the Clinical Scholars Program and later as chair of the Department of Medicine. Before joining GSK, Dr. Horwitz was chair of medicine at Stanford University and dean of Case Western Reserve Medical School. He is an elected member of the IOM of the National Academy of Sciences; the American Society for Clinical Investigation; the American Epidemiological Society; and the Association of American Physicians (he was president in 2010). He was a member of the Advisory Committee to the NIH director, under both Elias Zerhouni and Francis Collins. Dr. Horwitz served on the American

Board of Internal Medicine and was chairman in 2003. He is a master of the American College of Physicians.

Jeffrey P. Kahn, Ph.D., M.P.H., is the inaugural Robert Henry Levi and Ryda Hecht Levi Professor of Bioethics and Public Policy at the Johns Hopkins Berman Institute of Bioethics and is professor in the Department of Health Policy and Management in the Johns Hopkins University Bloomberg School of Public Health. Prior to joining the faculty at Johns Hopkins in 2011, Dr. Kahn was director of the Center for Bioethics and the Maas Family Endowed Chair in Bioethics at the University of Minnesota, positions he held from 1996 to 2011. Earlier in his career, Dr. Kahn was director of the graduate program in bioethics and assistant professor of bioethics at the Medical College of Wisconsin (1992–1996), and from April 1994 to October 1995 he was associate director of the White House Advisory Committee on Human Radiation Experiments. Dr. Kahn works in a variety of areas of bioethics, exploring the intersection of ethics and public health policy, including research ethics, ethics and genetics, and ethical issues in public health. He has served on numerous state and federal advisory panels and speaks nationally and internationally on a range of bioethics topics. He has published more than 125 articles in the bioethics and medical literature and is a coeditor of the widely used text *Contemporary Issues in Bioethics*, now in its eighth edition. From 1998 to 2002 he wrote the biweekly column "Ethics Matters" for CNN.com. Dr. Kahn earned his B.A. in microbiology from UC Los Angeles, his M.P.H. from Johns Hopkins University, and his Ph.D. in philosophy/bioethics from Georgetown University.

Robin T. Kelley, Ph.D., M.S.W., is evaluation manager at the National AIDS Minority Council. Dr. Kelley received a doctorate in public and community health from the University of Maryland and a master's degree in social work from Columbia University. She has recently received a Fulbright Senior Specialist Award to train faculty who teach front-line health care workers in Zanzibar. She has worked for more than 18 years as a program and evaluation consultant, behavioral scientist, program developer, program director, and evaluator for community-based health organizations focused on vulnerable populations in the United States and abroad. Dr. Kelley has taught women's health and human rights at Georgetown University and women's health at George Washington University and at the Washington Center for Internships and Academic Seminars.

Margaret McCabe, Ph.D., R.N., P.N.P., is the director of nursing research for medicine patient services at Boston Children's Hospital. In this role she educates and mentors staff in the conduct of evidence-based practice (EBP) and clinical research. At the same time Dr. McCabe maintains her own program of research that focuses on using a biobehavioral framework to better understand the symptom of fatigue in children. Dr. McCabe holds a faculty appointment at Harvard Medical School and has taught undergraduate and graduate nursing courses at several schools of nursing. Her teaching most often focuses on the basic elements of research design for clinical inquiry emphasizing the process of developing clinically relevant and feasible research questions. She completed post-doctoral training at the Harvard School of Public Health and Yale School of Nursing. Dr. McCabe is a past-president and founding member of the International Association for Clinical Research Nurses. Through the course of her nursing career Dr. McCabe has worked in roles providing direct patient care, managing care units for patients participating in research protocols and developing and implementing clinical research protocols. Dr. McCabe has been involved in research activities taking place in a range of settings from the laboratory to the community.

Edith A. Perez, M.D., is the deputy director-at-large for the Mayo Clinic Cancer Center in Florida, group vice-chair of the Alliance for Clinical Trials in Oncology, director of the Breast Program, and the Serene M. and Frances C. Durling Professor of Medicine at Mayo Medical School. She is a cancer specialist and an internationally known translational researcher at the Mayo Clinic. Her roles extend nationally, including positions within Mayo Clinic, the American Association for Cancer Research, the American Society of Clinical Oncology, and the National Cancer Institute. Dr. Perez has developed, and is involved in, a wide range of clinical trials exploring the use of new therapeutic agents for the treatment and prevention of breast cancer. She leads and has helped develop basic research studies to evaluate the role of genetic markers in the development and aggressiveness of breast cancer. She has written more than 550 research articles and abstracts in journals and books. Dr. Perez is frequently invited to lecture at national and international meetings and serves on the editorial boards of multiple academic journals. A select list of awards Dr. Perez has received includes the Breast Cancer Research Foundation Research Grant Award (1998–2013); Horizon Achievement Award in Cancer Research (2002); Mayo Clinic Outstanding Faculty

Award (2002 and 2004); North Florida Hispanic of the Year Award (2003); Mayo Clinic Distinguished Educator Award (2003); Honorary Doctorate of Letters, University of North Florida (2006); Mayo Clinic Distinguished Investigator (2007); Florida State Biomedical Research Advisory Council (BRAC) (2009–2012); Alpha Omega Alpha Honor Medical Society (2009); Mayo Clinic Outstanding Course Director (2009); EVE Award for Lifetime Achievement (2011); NFL Hispanic Heritage Leadership Award (2011); and 1 of the 75 Most Influential People in Jacksonville HealthCare from Jacksonville's *904 Magazine* (2012).

Clifford J. Rosen, M.D., is senior scientist at Maine Medical Center's Research Institute. He is the former director of the Maine Center for Osteoporosis Research and Education, an affiliate of St. Joseph Hospital and a center that he started more than 20 years ago. He previously conducted more than 20 NIH- and pharmaceutical-sponsored clinical research trials, as well as currently overseeing three investigator-initiated, NIH-funded translational projects and one program project. He is past president of the American Society of Bone and Mineral Research (2002–2003) and served 5 years as the first editor-in-chief of the *Journal of Clinical Densitometry* as well as associate editor of the *Journal of Bone and Mineral Research* and the *Journal of Clinical Endocrinology and Metabolism.* Dr. Rosen is currently the editor-in-chief of *The Primer on the Metabolic Bone Diseases and Disorders of Mineral Metabolism* and previously served a 4-year term on the advisory council for the National Institute of Arthritis and Musculoskeletal and Skin Diseases and a 10-year term on the FDA's Endocrinologic and Metabolic Drugs Advisory Committee. He is also a member of several professional societies, including the Endocrine Society, the American Society of Bone and Mineral Research, and the American Federation of Clinical Research. Dr. Rosen is a professor of medicine at Tufts University School of Medicine and currently studies the role of insulin-like growth factors, bone marrow adiposity, and stem cells in skeletal remodeling. His work includes more than 325 manuscripts in a variety of journals, including *Nature Medicine,* the *New England Journal of Medicine,* and the *Proceedings of the National Academy of Sciences of the United States of America.* Dr. Rosen received his medical degree from the State University of New York, Syracuse.